I0428299

GREEN & NATURAL

Hair, Lip, & Nail Care Recipes

Copyright 2011

Pippen

Library of Congress -in-Publication Data
September 2011

All rights reserved. No part of this book or applicable additions may be reproduced in any form or by any means.
Printed in the United States of America

10 9 8 7 6 5 4 3 2 1

The recipes in this book are all made with easily obtained ingredients that are generally accepted to be safe and effective.

Individual reactions to the contained ingredients can vary. It is not possible to predict how any individual will react to a particular recipe, treatment, or ingredient.

As with any personal care product common sense should be used when creating these recipes. The reader should consult a qualified physician before using any ingredient or created recipe in this book.

The enclosed materials are for informational purposes only and the reader accepts all responsibility for determining the effectiveness and usefulness of all included items. Neither the author nor the publisher accepts and liability neither for the actions of the reader nor for any reactions caused by the use of the contents and ingredients.

To obtain information or inquire about availability please write to Director, PO Box 1, Hollidaysburg, PA 16648

NOTICE

The enclosed materials are copyrighted materials. Federal law prohibits the unauthorized reproduction, distribution or exhibit of the materials. The materials contained within this publication are distributed for personal use. Violations of copyright law will be prosecuted.

From the US Code Collection – Violation of Copyright is a Criminal Offense

Criminal Infringement—Any person who infringes a copyright willfully either

    (1)   **for the purpose of commercial advantage or private financial gain or**

    (2)   **by the reproduction or distribution, including by electronic means during any 180-day period, of 1 or more copyrighted works, shall be punished as provided under section 2319 of title 18, United States Code.**

In General.—except as otherwise provided by this title, an infringer of copyright is liable for

    (1)   **the copyright owner's actual damages and any additional profits of the Infringer**

    (2)   **statutory damages**

Violations of copyright will be prosecuted as allowed under law.

GREEN & NATURAL

Hair, Lip, & Nail Care Recipes

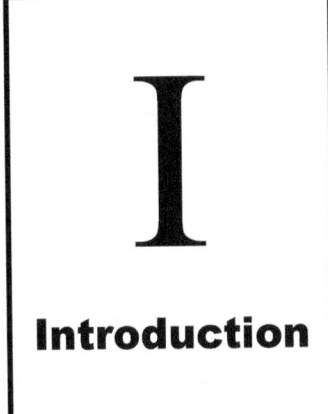

I

Introduction

A walk down the personal care product aisles in your local store can be a lot of fun. There seems to be a product available for just about any need, issue, or desire. Even with such a huge selection, when you start going through each one, you will often find that the exact product you need just is not there.

The products in the personal care aisle are created for everyone, not for the individual. You often know exactly what you want and the results you desire, but because each of us is different with slightly different needs and preferences these products never quite measure up to our expectations.

There is a solution. A cost effective, natural solution customized just for you. Many people do not realize that with key ingredients easily obtained from your grocery store, yard, and kitchen, they can make an entire hair and nail product line of their own. Better yet, they can make them with fewer unnatural additives. By following simple recipes, a lot like those in a cook book, you can create your very own hair and nail care line. This line will be customized to meet your exact needs. Best yet, this line costs only pennies compared to those items you find in the personal care aisle!

The recipes and alternative ingredient list in this book will help you start creating a hair and nail care line custom suited to your wants, preference, and needs.

You can have the fun and excitement of creating your very own shampoos, conditioners, and treatments.

> You can save hundreds of dollars a year by creating the exact products that you and your family want and need for a fraction of the money you will pay for pre-prepared products.

> You can address personal issues, problems, and needs in a way that is focused entirely on you.

> You can create a healthier life for your family by using all-natural ingredients.

> You can even start your own line of personal care products to share with friends, family, and the world!

Each chapter of the book will provide you with some recipes that are the core products you will use to fill your personal care cabinets. Each of these can be expanded and customized to suit your personal needs. The appendix includes an ingredient list that gives a brief summary of the expected benefit of each ingredient. This list provides you with a basis for customizing each recipe, and beginning to create your own brand new products!

This book is all about experimenting to determine what is best for you! The recipes included are all customizable by exchanging the ingredients I use with the ones you prefer from the ingredient list. I change the recipes continuously to suit the time of year, my personal preferences or even which member of my family is likely to use a particular product.

Remember, no two people have exactly the same needs. Each year I try to make a personal care gift pack for each person in my extended family. These gifts are fantastic for holidays and special events since they are created especially for the person receiving the package! These personalized products would cost you hundreds of dollars at a customized shop and still not provide the same benefits as those items you create in your own kitchen.

Now you can have those costly, personalized products that you see in the store but are unwilling to try or that you do buy, much to the detriment of your wallet! You can have these products for just pennies and now, you can provide these same products for you friends and family!

CHAPTER 1

Shampoos & Washes

Beautiful hair starts with clean hair. The shampoo that you use really does make a difference.

I have thick hair that can go from straight to curly depending on the treatments that I use. This can be great as long as I start planning how I will wear my hair before I ever step into the shower. If I don't my hair just goes to frizz no matter what post shower products I try to use to tame it.

Everyone has a hair story similar to mine. By creating custom hair care products developed specifically toward your hair type, preferred style, and special issues you can have perfect hair every day!

Salon hair treatments almost always work as expected but they can be costly and usually contain chemicals that can do more long term harm than one days worth of beautiful hair is worth.

The good news is that I have not yet found a salon product that can not be duplicated using all natural ingredients. Better yet, the cost of each product is a fraction of the companion salon products. In fact, most of these recipes cost less to create than the bargain products found at any mass merchant!

Each recipe in this chapter defines hair care for specific needs. You may find the perfect product right here on these pages. If not, you can refer to the optional ingredient list and start making simple changes to the recipe to create the products perfect for your hair care needs.

Before you begin customizing your hair care recipes, you should understand that there is a difference between home made shampoo and commercial shampoo. Commercial shampoo uses chemical additives that help create sudsy bubbles. This makes most people feel like their shampoo is really working. These chemical additives are not necessary to clean hair.

Give yourself a little bit of time to get used to the lower quantity of suds in natural shampoo or use a foaming additive from the ingredient list to help your sudsing action. Rest assured suds or no, these shampoos do a nice job cleansing the hair.

Shampoo is just a cleanser. Almost every recipe I use starts with one of these basic shampoo recipes. I mix up a huge batch of basic shampoo and then customize the added ingredients toward the season, hair type, and styling goals of the person who will use the shampoo.

Normal Hair Shampoo Base

This is a nice shampoo for normal hair or hair that is not too oily or too dry.

- ½ cup   Water
- 1 cup   Liquid Castile Soap
- 1 tsp   Palm Kernel Oil
- 1 tsp   Jojoba Oil

Mix the ingredients

Pour into a clean squeeze bottle

Use in place of your regular shampoo

Use this shampoo as a base for custom blending for specific hair care needs

Normal to Dry Hair Shampoo Base

This is a nice shampoo for normal to slightly dry hair care.

- ➤ 1 cup   Water

- ➤ 1 cup   Liquid Castile Soap

- ➤ 1 tsp   Aloe Vera Gel

- ➤ 1 tsp   Jojoba Oil

- ➤ 1 tbsp   Palm Kernel Oil

Mix the ingredients

Pour into a clean squeeze bottle

Use in place of your regular shampoo

Use this shampoo as a base for custom blending for specific hair care needs

Extremely Dry or Treated Hair Shampoo Base

This is a slightly more moisturizing shampoo for dry hair care.

- ➢ ½ cup   Water

- ➢ 1 cup   Liquid Castile Soap

- ➢ 2 tbsp   Aloe Vera Gel

- ➢ 1 tbsp   Vegetable Glycerin

- ➢ 1 tbsp   Jojoba Oil

- ➢ 1 tbsp   Palm Kernel Oil

Mix the ingredients

Pour into a clean squeeze bottle

Use in place of your regular shampoo

Use this shampoo as a base for custom blending for specific hair care needs

Normal to Slightly Oily Hair Shampoo Base

This is a nice shampoo for oily days. I find it a bit drying for my hair but it is perfect for my husband and son. If you hair is lightly oily, this is a better alternative shampoo base.

> - 2 cup   Hot Water
> - ½ cup   Borax Powder
> - ½ cup   Liquid Glycerin
> - 1 tsp   Jojoba Oil
> - 1 tsp   Palm Kernel Oil

Dissolve borax powder in water

Stir in remaining ingredients

Pour into a clean squeeze bottle

Use in place of your regular shampoo

Use this shampoo as a base for custom blending for specific hair care needs

Oily Hair Shampoo Base

This is a nice shampoo for hair that tends more toward oily.

- ➤ 2 cup   Hot Water

- ➤ ½ cup   Borax Powder

- ➤ ½ cup   Liquid Glycerin

- ➤ 1 tbsp   Grapeseed Oil

- ➤ 1 tbsp   Palm Kernel Oil

- ➤ 2 tbsp   Apple Cider or White Vinegar

Dissolve borax powder in water

Stir in remaining ingredients

Pour into a clean squeeze bottle

Use in place of your regular shampoo

Use this shampoo as a base for custom blending for specific hair care needs

These shampoo customizations are some of my favorites. Each one uses one of the four shampoo base recipes. You should experiment with different bases and ingredients to find the combination that works best for you.

Moisture Infusing Shampoo

This is a wonderful moisturizing shampoo that I think adds just enough weight to keep my fly away hair in place.

- ➢ 1 cup   Shampoo Base Recipe of choice

             I recommend either:

             Normal to Dry Hair Shampoo Base

             Extremely Dry or Treated Hair Base

- ➢ ½ cup   Aloe Vera Gel

- ➢ 1 tsp   Liquid Glycerin

- ➢ 1 tsp   Jojoba Oil

- ➢ 1 tbsp   Coconut Oil

Blend all ingredients

Pour into a clean squeeze bottle

Use in place of your regular shampoo

Super Moisture Shampoo

This is a wonderful moisturizing shampoo that I think adds just enough weight to keep my fly away hair in place.

- ➤ 1 cup   Shampoo Base Recipe of choice

  I recommend either:

  Normal to Dry Hair Shampoo Base

  Extremely Dry or Treated Hair

- ➤ ½ cup   Aloe Vera Gel
- ➤ 2 tbsp   Meadowfoam Seed Oil

Blend all ingredients

Pour into a clean squeeze bottle

Use in place of your regular shampoo

Strengthening Shampoo

Regardless of your hair type, we all need a little strength in our hair now and then. When my hair starts to look damaged from the sun, wind, and styling I love to use this in combination with a strengthening pre-treatment and deep conditioner.

- ➤ 1 cup   Shampoo Base of Choice

    I recommend

    Normal to Dry Hair Shampoo Base

    Normal to Slightly Oily Hair Base

- ➤ ½ cup   Hot Water

- ➤ ¼ cup   Gelatin

- ➤ 2 tsp   Rosehip Seed Oil

Blend all ingredients

Pour into a clean squeeze bottle

Use in place of your regular shampoo

Repair Shampoo

Regardless of your hair type, we all need a little strength in our hair now and then. When my hair starts to look damaged from the sun, wind, and styling I love to use this in combination with a strengthening pre-treatment and deep conditioner.

- ➤ 1 cup   Shampoo Base of Choice

  I recommend

  Normal to Dry Hair Shampoo Base

  Normal to Slightly Oily Hair Base

- ➤ ½ cup   Hot Water
- ➤ ¼ cup   Gelatin
- ➤ 1 tbsp   Colorless Henna
- ➤ 2 tbsp   Meadowfoam Seed Oil

Dissolve Gelatin and Henna in hot water

Add remaining ingredients

Blend well

Pour into a clean squeeze bottle

Use in place of your regular shampoo

Body Building Shampoo

Bouncy, full hair is something we all admire. This shampoo helps to thicken the hair while adding a nice luster.

- ➢ 1 cup   Shampoo Base of your choice

    I recommend

    Normal to Dry Hair Shampoo Base

    Normal to Slightly Oily Hair Base

- ➢ 1 cup   Beer or Champagne – scent will diminish over time

- ➢ 2 tbsp   Wheat Protein

- ➢ 2 tbsp   Powdered Gelatin

Heat beer or champagne slightly

Dissolve wheat protein and gelatin in warmed liquid

Blend remaining ingredients

Pour into a clean squeeze bottle

Use in place of your regular shampoo

Hydrating Shampoo

Just like skin, hydration is critical to attractive, healthy hair that does what you want. This is a nice shampoo that leaves my hair well hydrated and looking great.

- ➤ 1 cup   Shampoo Base of your choice

                 I recommend

                 Normal to Dry Hair Shampoo Base

                 Normal to Slightly Oily Hair Base

- ➤ 2 tbsp   Powdered Gelatin
- ➤ ¼ cup   Hot Water
- ➤ 2 tbsp   Pure Honey
- ➤ 1 tbsp   Paw Paw Extract

Heat water

Dissolve gelatin in warmed liquid

Blend remaining ingredients

Pour into a clean squeeze bottle

Use in place of your regular shampoo

Anti Frizz Shampoo

Just like skin, hydration is critical to attractive, healthy hair that does what you want. This is a nice shampoo that leaves my hair well hydrated and looking great.

> 1 cup   Shampoo Base of your choice

              I recommend

              Normal to Dry Hair Shampoo Base

              Normal to Slightly Oily Hair Base

> 2 tbsp   Powdered Gelatin

> ¼ cup   Apple, Pear, or Berry Juice

> 2 tbsp   Wheat Germ

> 1 tbsp   Almond Oil

Heat water

Dissolve gelatin and wheat germ in warmed liquid

Blend remaining ingredients

Pour into a clean squeeze bottle

Use in place of your regular shampoo

Clarifying Shampoo – Oily Hair

Just like skin, hydration is critical to attractive, healthy hair that does what you want. This is a nice shampoo that leaves my hair well hydrated and looking great.

- ➢ 1 cup   Shampoo Base of your choice

  I recommend

  Normal to Dry Hair Shampoo Base

  Normal to Slightly Oily Hair Base

- ➢ 2 tbsp   Lemon Juice

- ➢ 2 tbsp   Pineapple Juice

Blend ingredients

Pour into a clean squeeze bottle

Use in place of your regular shampoo

Clarifying Shampoo – Normal Hair

Just like skin, hydration is critical to attractive, healthy hair that does what you want. This is a nice shampoo that leaves my hair well hydrated and looking great.

> - 1 cup   Shampoo Base of your choice

    I recommend

    Normal to Dry Hair Shampoo Base

    Normal to Slightly Oily Hair Base

> - 2 tbsp   Orange Flower Water

> - 1 tbsp   Jojoba Oil

> - ¼ tsp   Baking Soda

Heat water

Dissolve gelatin in warmed liquid

Blend remaining ingredients

Pour into a clean squeeze bottle

Use in place of your regular shampoo

Dandruff Control Shampoo

Dandruff is dead skin. Everyone sheds skin cells from every part of their body everyday, including the scalp. Most of us never noticed. Dandruff can sometimes be caused by these skin cells failing to release. Keeping your scalp clean and well hydrated is the best solution to a build up of dead skin cells.

Dandruff can also occur when your scalp becomes extremely dry. Using a deep conditioning treatment and an oil infusing set will help control dry skin on the scalp in the same way lotions control dry skin on your body.

Dandruff can also be a result of microscopic fungus living on your scalp. The dandruff treatments included in the chapters of this book help to eliminate this fungus and restore your scalp to a clean, healthy condition.

You should always consult with a physician before using any medicinal treatments and side effects vary by individuals.

Serious conditions of the scalp should always be treated by a physician. Less severe cases may respond well to home treatment.

Daily Dandruff Shampoo

This is a nice shampoo that helps give your hair a shiny luster while reducing dandruff.

- ➢ ¼ cup — Hot Water

- ➢ 2 tbsp — Ginger Root

    (Fresh is better, but you can use dried)

Boil the water

Steep ginger root in hot water for 60-90 minutes until you have a very strong brew

- ➢ ½ cup — Normal to Dry Hair Shampoo Base

- ➢ 1 tsp — Lemon Juice

- ➢ 1 tbsp — Sesame Seed Oil

Blend remaining ingredients

Pour into a clean squeeze bottle

Massage into your scalp

Allow shampoo to sit on scalp 5-15 minutes

Repeat daily

Hair Loss Daily Shampoo

1 tsp   burdock root

¼ cup   warm water

Allow to steep 30 minutes

Strain roots   Can use Bur Oil in replacement

Add

1 tbsp   powdered ginger root

1 tbsp   powdered lemon balm

1 tbsp   birch bark oil

1 tbsp   black seed oil

1 tbsp   muira puama

1 tsp   lemon juice

20 drops   saw palmetto oil

Incorporate into 1 cup shampoo base

Do not use if you are on blood thinning medication, anti-coagulants or have a disorder related to blood
Do not use if you are pregnant or nursing
Do not use if you are unable to use aspirin
Not for use on children
For EXTERNAL use only

Fast Hair Growth Shampoo

1 tsp   burdock root

2 tbsp   apache plume

½ cup   boiling water

Steep 30 minutes

Add

2 tbsp   rosemary tincture

Incorporate into

1 cup   shampoo base

Use daily

Do not use if you are pregnant or nursing

CHAPTER

2

Color Enhancers

Nothing looks better than well toned and highlighted hair. Unless you are trying to completely change the look of your hair, you can use color enhancers to make subtle changes to the color of your hair that look completely natural.

Color enhancers use your natural tone and add subtle colorants that give it a whole new look.

I like to use a combination of shampoo, rinses, and conditioner to speed the process and keep my highlights, or lowlights, looking fresh. You can choose to use only one or a combination of the color enhancing products depending on how deep and fast you want to make the change.

Depending on your color preferences, consider using different enhancers for different times of the year. I have very dark hair that tends toward auburn when I get enough sun. I use the brunette enhancers in the winter but switch red in the warmer months.

Blond Color Enhancing Shampoo

If you have light brown to blond hair and want a natural daily enhancer, this shampoo is perfect. Each time you wash, the shampoo will enhance your natural colors and help promote a lovely blond glow. Use with color rinses and color enhancing conditioners for best results.

- ➢ 1 cup   Shampoo Base of your choice

                              I recommend

                              Normal to Dry Hair Shampoo Base

                              Normal to Slightly Oily Hair Base

- ➢ 2 tbsp   Lemon Juice

- ➢ ½ tsp   Sesame Seed Oil

- ➢ ¼ cup   Hot Water

- ➢ 2 tbsp   Chamomile
                              (You can use 2 teabags if necessary)

Boil water and chamomile

Allow to steep at least 30 minutes until you have a strong brew

Blend remaining ingredients

Pour into a clean squeeze bottle

Use in place of your regular shampoo

Alternative Blond Color Enhancing Shampoo

If you have light brown to blond hair and want a natural daily enhancer, this shampoo is perfect. Each time you wash, the shampoo will enhance your natural colors and help promote a lovely blond glow. Use with color rinses and color enhancing conditioners for best results.

- ➢ 1 cup   Shampoo Base of your choice

                   I recommend

                   Normal to Dry Hair Shampoo Base

                   Normal to Slightly Oily Hair Base

- ➢ 1 cup   Boiling Water
- ➢ 2 tbsp   Calendula
- ➢ 2 tbsp   Rhubarb

Boil water and herbs

Allow to steep at least 30 minutes until you have a strong brew

Blend remaining ingredients

Pour into a clean squeeze bottle

Use in place of your regular shampoo

Dark Color Enhancing Shampoo

If you have light brown to dark hair and want a natural daily enhancer, this shampoo is perfect. Each time you wash, the shampoo will enhance your natural colors and help deepen your lovely dark locks.

- ➤ 1 cup   Shampoo Base of your choice

                I recommend

                Normal to Dry Hair Shampoo Base
                Normal to Slightly Oily Hair Base

- ➤ 1 cup   Boiling Water

- ➤ 2 tbsp   Fresh Rosemary
                (You may use 2 teabags if preferred)

- ➤ 2 tbsp   Cloves

- ➤ 1 tbsp   Dark Tea Leaves

Boil water and herbs

Allow to steep at least 30 minutes until you have a strong brew

Blend remaining ingredients

Pour into a clean squeeze bottle

Use in place of your regular shampoo

Alternative Dark Color Enhancing Shampoo

If you have light brown to dark hair and want a natural daily enhancer, this shampoo is perfect. Each time you wash, the shampoo will enhance your natural colors and help deepen your lovely dark locks.

> 1 cup   Shampoo Base of your choice

                   I recommend

                   Normal to Dry Hair Shampoo Base

                   Normal to Slightly Oily Hair Base

> 1 cup   Boiling Water

> 2 tbsp   Cinnamon

> 2 tbsp   Rhubarb

Boil water and herbs

Allow to steep at least 30 minutes until you have a strong brew

Blend remaining ingredients

Pour into a clean squeeze bottle

Use in place of your regular shampoo

Red Color Enhancing Shampoo

Whether you have blond, red, brown, or black and want a natural red tone added through a daily enhancer, this shampoo is perfect. Each time you wash, the shampoo will enhance your natural colors and help deepen your lovely dark locks.

> ➢ 1 cup   Shampoo Base of your choice
>
>   I recommend
>
>   Normal to Dry Hair Shampoo Base
>
>   Normal to Slightly Oily Hair Base

> ➢ 1 cup   Boiling Water
>
> ➢ 2 tbsp   Hibiscus Oil
>
> ➢ 2 tbsp   Cinnamon Bark

Boil water and herbs

Allow to steep at least 30 minutes until you have a strong brew

Blend remaining ingredients

Pour into a clean squeeze bottle

Use in place of your regular shampoo

Gray Enhancing Shampoo

If you have gray hair and want a natural daily enhancer, this shampoo is perfect. Each time you wash, the shampoo will enhance your natural colors and help deepen your lovely dark locks.

- ➢ 1 cup   Shampoo Base of your choice

  I recommend

  Normal to Dry Hair Shampoo Base

  Normal to Slightly Oily Hair Base

- ➢ 1 cup   Boiling Water

- ➢ 2 tbsp   Sage

- ➢ 2 tbsp   Thyme

- ➢ 2 tbsp   Rosemary

Boil water and herbs

Allow to steep at least 30 minutes until you have a strong brew

Blend remaining ingredients

Pour into a clean squeeze bottle

Use in place of your regular shampoo

Herbal Hair Rinse

A post shampoo and conditioner hair rinse is an excellent way to reduce product build up, tone your hair, and highlight your color at the same time.

These products rely on herbs

You can purchase ready made herb tea bags or you can make your own. I like to buy fresh herbs and use them as is or dry them myself.

How to Make a Homemade Tea Bag

You will need a tea ball or make a homemade teabag for this recipe

Cut a coffee filter into rectangles approximately 1 ½ inch x 2 inches

Fold the rectangle in half length wise

Place the herb of your choice in the center of the tea bag

Close fold over herbs

Turn ends of bag toward the center

I use a small stapler to close the bag and add the string or thread

Use as you would your regular tea bag

Blond Toning Hair Rinse

One of the most effective hair dyes I have found is to use a gradual wash in toning rinse. Use this rinse each day after you shampoo and condition. Allow to dry on the hair.

- ➤ 2 cups   Distilled water

- ➤ 2 tbsp   Rhubarb

- ➤ 4 tbsp   Chamomile

Bring the water to a boil

Steep herbs in the water at least 90 minutes or until you have achieved a strong brew

- ➤ 2 tbsp   White Vinegar

Add vinegar

Pour in to a clean pump container

Work through hair after your shampoo and conditioner

Do not rinse

Your hair will have a conditioned luster throughout the day

Brown Toning Hair Rinse

One of the most effective hair dyes I have found is to use a gradual wash in toning rinse. Use this rinse each day after you shampoo and condition. Allow to dry on the hair.

- ➢ 2 cups   Distilled water

- ➢ 2 tbsp   Lavender Oil

- ➢ 4 tbsp   Rosemary Leaves

Bring the water to a boil

Steep herbs in the water at least 90 minutes or until you have achieved a strong brew

- ➢ 2 tbsp   White Vinegar

Add vinegar

Pour in to a clean pump container

Work through hair after your shampoo and conditioner

Do not rinse

Your hair will have a conditioned luster throughout the day

Red Toning Hair Rinse

One of the most effective hair dyes I have found is to use a gradual wash in toning rinse. Use this rinse each day after you shampoo and condition. Allow to dry on the hair.

- ➢ 2 cups   Distilled water
- ➢ 2 tbsp   Hibiscus
- ➢ 4 tbsp   Rhubarb

Bring the water to a boil

Steep herbs in the water at least 90 minutes or until you have achieved a strong brew

- ➢ 2 tbsp   White Vinegar

Add vinegar

Pour in to a clean pump container

Work through hair after your shampoo and conditioner

Do not rinse

Your hair will have a conditioned luster throughout the day

Daily Conditioning Treatment for Blond Hair

One of the most effective hair dyes I have found is to use a gradual daily agent. Use this conditioner in conjunction with your color enhancing shampoo.

- ➢ ¼ cup   Distilled water

- ➢ 1 tbsp   Rhubarb

- ➢ 1 tbsp   Chamomile

Bring the water to a boil

Steep herbs in the water at least 90 minutes or until you have achieved a strong brew

- ➢ ¼ cup   Aloe Vera Gel

- ➢ 1 tsp   Vegetable Glycerin

- ➢ 1 tsp   Almond Oil

Blend remaining ingredients

Pour into a clean squeeze bottle

Use in place of your regular conditioner

Do not rinse this entirely out of the hair for the best toning effect

Daily Conditioning Treatment for Dark Hair

One of the most effective hair dyes I have found is to use a gradual daily agent. Use this conditioner in conjunction with your color enhancing shampoo.

> - ½ cup   Distilled water
> - 2 tbsp   Lavender Oil
> - 4 tbsp   Rosemary Leaves

Bring the water to a boil

Steep herbs in the water at least 90 minutes or until you have achieved a strong brew

> - ¼ cup   Aloe Vera Gel
> - 1 tsp   Vegetable Glycerin
> - 1 tsp   Almond Oil

Blend remaining ingredients

Pour into a clean squeeze bottle

Use in place of your regular conditioner

Do not rinse this entirely out of the hair for the best toning effect

Daily Conditioning Treatment for Red Hair

One of the most effective hair dyes I have found is to use a gradual daily agent. Use this conditioner in conjunction with your color enhancing shampoo.

- ➢ ½ cup   Distilled water

- ➢ 2 tbsp   Hibiscus

- ➢ 4 tbsp   Rhubarb

Bring the water to a boil

Steep herbs in the water at least 90 minutes or until you have achieved a strong brew

- ➢ ¼ cup   Aloe Vera Gel

- ➢ 1 tsp   Vegetable Glycerin

- ➢ 1 tsp   Almond Oil

Blend remaining ingredients

Pour into a clean squeeze bottle

Use in place of your regular conditioner

Do not rinse this entirely out of the hair for the best toning effect

Daily Conditioning Treatment for Gray Hair

One of the most effective hair dyes I have found is to use a gradual daily agent. Use this conditioner in conjunction with your color enhancing shampoo.

- ½ cup Distilled water
- 2 tbsp Sage
- 2 tbsp Thyme
- 2 tbsp Rosemary

Boil water and herbs

Allow to steep at least 30 minutes until you have a strong brew

- ¼ cup Aloe Vera Gel
- 1 tsp Vegetable Glycerin
- 1 tsp Almond Oil

Blend remaining ingredients

Pour into a clean squeeze bottle

Use in place of your regular conditioner

Do not rinse this entirely out of the hair for the best toning effect

CHAPTER 3

Hot Oil Treatments

Whether your hair is dry and damaged from too much styling, overstressed by life and environment, or just in need a little TLC time, hot oil treatments can work wonders for the health of your hair.

I like to use a hot oil treatment once a month or so during normal times. If my hair is exposed to too much sun or chlorine, overstressed from styling, or just being a problem, I use the treatments once a week until I have happy healthy hair again.

These are my favorite treatments, but nearly any oil that is compatible with your hair and skin can be a great hot oil treatment. You should review the optional ingredient listing and experiment to find the perfect oil for your needs.

Moisture Infusing Hot Oil Treatment

This is nice for moderately to extremely dry hair. I also like to use it in the winter when there is just not enough moisture to go around.

- ➤ 1 tbsp   Almond Oil

- ➤ 2 tbsp   Sesame Seed Oil

- ➤ ¼ tsp   Avocado Oil

Place oils in a Dixie sized cup

Blend well

Fill a bowl with very hot water. I like to heat it almost to boiling in the microwave

Place oil cup in the bowl of hot water

Allow the oils to heat while you lightly moisten your hair

Apply the warmed oil mixture to your hair paying close attention to the ends

Wrap your hair in plastic

Wait 20-30 minutes

Wash the hair as usual

Dry & Damaged Hair Hot Oil Treatment

We all style our hair. We use products. We do damage. This is a fantastic treatment that helps heal the shaft of the hair, repairing damage, and leaving hair looking and feeling great.

> - 1 tbsp   Meadowfoam Seed Oil

> - 1 tbsp   Nettle Leaf

> - ½ tbsp   Rosehip Seed Oil

Place oils in a Dixie sized cup

Blend well

Fill a bowl with very hot water. I like to heat it almost to boiling in the microwave

Place oil cup in the bowl of hot water

Allow the oils to heat while you lightly moisten your hair

Apply the warmed oil mixture to your hair paying close attention to the ends

Wrap your hair in plastic

Wait 20-30 minutes

Wash the hair as usual

Hydrating Heat Treatment

Just like skin, healthy hair need so to be hydrated to look its best. I like this treatment when my hair starts to look a little dull and flat. It adds a fantastic luster while attracting and holding moisture.

- ➤ 1 tbsp   Vegetable Glycerin

- ➤ 1 tbsp   Honey

- ➤ 1 tsp   Paw Paw Oil

Place oils in a Dixie sized cup

Blend well

Fill a bowl with very hot water. I like to heat it almost to boiling in the microwave

Place oil cup in the bowl of hot water

Allow the oils to heat while you lightly moisten your hair

Apply the warmed oil mixture to your hair paying close attention to the ends

Wrap your hair in plastic

Wait 20-30 minutes

Wash the hair as usual

Anti-Frizz Hot Oil Treatment

Frizz is the biggest problem that I have with my hair. I have naturally wavy hair that sometimes likes to go straight. Most days it seems like it cannot decide what it wants so it just opts for frizz. This is one of the best treatments I have found to stop frizz before it has the chance to start.

- ➢ 1 tbsp   Almond Oil

- ➢ 1 tbsp   Wheat Germ

- ➢ 1 tbsp   Aloe Vera Gel

Place oils in a Dixie sized cup

Blend well

Fill a bowl with very hot water. I like to heat it almost to boiling in the microwave

Place oil cup in the bowl of hot water

Allow the oils to heat while you lightly moisten your hair

Apply the warmed oil mixture to your hair paying close attention to the ends

Wrap your hair in plastic

Wait 20-30 minutes

Wash the hair as usual

Dandruff Control Hot Oil Treatment

Some dandruff is caused by an over dry scalp while other dandruff is caused by microscopic fungi living on the scalp. This hot oil treatment combines intense moisture with antibacterial components to help address both problems.

- ➢ 1 tbsp   Lavender Oil

- ➢ 1 tbsp   Rosemary Oil

- ➢ 1 tbsp   Lemon Oil

Place oils in a Dixie sized cup

Blend well

Fill a bowl with very hot water. I like to heat it almost to boiling in the microwave

Place oil cup in the bowl of hot water

Allow the oils to heat while you lightly moisten your hair

Apply the warmed oil mixture to your hair paying close attention to the ends

Wrap your hair in plastic

Wait 20-30 minutes

Wash the hair as usual

CHAPTER 4

Conditioner

Conditioner is important for healthy hair. Most conditioners are simply an oil and cream mixture. Homemade conditioners will usually be oilier and less like a lotion than what you are used to from commercial products.

Commercial products contain a great many unnecessary additives. Home made conditioners tend to be more condensed. You will use less of the home made conditioners because it has fewer additives and fillers.

Once you get used to the texture and application differences, you will find that or the natural conditioners you make at home are far more effective than their commercial counterparts.

Conditioners are very specific to the user and each recipe must be custom blended to fit the end goal. These are some of my favorite conditioner recipes. Each one is a good daily conditioner.

Daily Conditioner
Dry or Damaged Hair

This is a heavier conditioner that helps to coat and protect dry hair while repairing damage. I use this when to help offset the damage caused by styling products.

- ➢ 3 tbsp   Jojoba Oil

- ➢ 1 tbsp   Sesame Seed Oil

- ➢ 2 tbsp   Rosehip Seed Oil

- ➢ ½ cup   Aloe Vera Gel

Blend all ingredients

Pour into a clean dry container

Massage into your hair and scalp

Rinse and repeat as needed

Alternative Daily Conditioner
Dry or Damaged Hair

This is a heavier conditioner that helps to coat and protect dry hair while repairing damage. I use this when to help offset the damage caused by styling products.

- ➢ 1 tbsp   Coconut Oil

- ➢ 1 tbsp   Sesame Seed Oil

- ➢ ½ cup   Aloe Vera Gel

- ➢ 2 tbsp   Meadowfoam Seed Oil

- ➢ 1 tbsp   Colorless Henna

- ➢ 4 tbsp   Warm Water

Heat water

Dissolve henna powder in warm water

Blend remaining ingredients

Pour into a clean dry container

Massage into your hair and scalp

Rinse and repeat as needed

Daily Conditioner
Normal to Slightly Dry Hair

This is a nice conditioner if you hair is normal or normal to dry. It gives a nice soft feel to the hair without too much weight.

- ¼ cup   Aloe Vera Gel

- 1 tsp   Vegetable Glycerin

- 1 tsp   Almond Oil

Blend ingredients

Pour into a clean dry container

Massage into your hair and scalp

Rinse and repeat as needed

Daily Conditioner
Normal Hair

I like this conditioner for normal hair. It gives a nice shine and light hydration without adding too much oil.

- ➤ 1 tsp   Liquid Glycerin

- ➤ 1 tbsp   Paw Paw Oil

- ➤ ¼ cup   Pear, Apple, or Berry Juice

- ➤ ¼ cup   Aloe Vera Gel

Blend ingredients

Pour into a clean dry container

Massage into your hair and scalp

Rinse and repeat as needed

Daily Conditioner
Normal to Lightly Oily Hair

My hair gets a little too oily at the scalp in the summer months. I like to use this to give my hair body while minimizing any potential oily residue.

- ➢ ½ cup   Aloe Vera Gel

- ➢ 2 tbsp   Pineapple Juice

- ➢ 2 tbsp   Jojoba Oil

Blend ingredients

Pour into a clean dry container

Massage into your hair and scalp

Rinse and repeat as needed

Daily Conditioner
Oily Hair

Using oils on oily hair seems counter productive in theory but all hair needs good, easily absorbed oil to promote health and protect it from the environment. Oily hair needs to have surface oils reduced while infusing it with easily absorbed health.

- ➢ ¼ cup   Aloe Vera Gel
- ➢ 2 tsp   Grape Seed Oil
- ➢ 1 tsp   Jojoba Oil

Blend ingredients

Pour into a clean dry container

Massage into your hair and scalp

Rinse and repeat as needed

Hydrating Conditioner

Moisture is important for beautiful hair, but just like any part of your body, hair craves hydration. This is actually my daily curly hair conditioner because it helps attract moisture and keeps hair well hydrated and healthy.

- ➤ ½ cup   Berry, Pear, or Apple Juice

- ➤ 1 tbsp   Unflavored Gelatin

- ➤ 2 tsp   Honey Powder

- ➤ 2 tbsp   Paw Paw Oil

Heat the juice until it is warmer than room temperature

Stir in gelatin and honey powder

Add oil

Blend well

Pour into a clean dry container

Massage into your hair and scalp

Rinse and repeat as needed

Volumizing Conditioner

Thinning or very fine hair is so difficult to style. This is a nice thickening conditioner that will help build body and add bounce when used in conjunction with the volumizing shampoo and hair gel.

- ¼ cup   Beer

- 1 tbsp   Gelatin Powder

- 1 tbsp   Almond Oil

Heat the beer until it is warmer than room temperature

Stir in gelatin

Add oil

Blend well

Pour into a clean dry container

Massage into your hair and scalp

Rinse and repeat as needed

The smell of the beer will fade as you style your hair

Frizz Control Conditioner

Rainy season around my region has become all 4 seasons of the year. My hair is thick and tends to frizz easily if I do not treat it the right way. I love this as a frizz control component. It helps tame fly away hair and minimize frizz even on the most humid days.

- ➤ ¼ cup   Cocoa Butter

- ➤ ¼ cup   Aloe Vera Gel

- ➤ 1 tsp   Almond Oil

- ➤ ¼ cup   Pear, Apple, or Berry Juice

Warm cocoa butter until it is thin enough to blend easily

Add remaining ingredients

Whip with a wire whisk

Pour into a clean dry tub or bottle

Massage into your hair and scalp

Rinse well

Dandruff Control Daily Conditioner

Some dandruff is caused by an over dry scalp while other dandruff is caused by microscopic fungi living on the scalp. This hot oil treatment combines intense moisture with antibacterial components to help address both problems.

- ➤ ¼ cup   Aloe Vera Gel

- ➤ 1 tbsp   Ginger Root Juice

- ➤ 2 tbsp   Sesame Seed Oil

Blend all remaining ingredients until you have a smooth mixture

Pour into a clean dry tub or bottle

Massage into your hair and scalp

Rinse well

Leave In Conditioner

Any of the daily conditioners can be converted to a leave in conditioner before you ever leave the shower.

> ➢ Wash and condition your hair as normal.

> ➢ Pour a pea sized amount of your preferred conditioner in the palm of your hand.

> ➢ Add approximately 1 tsp of water

> ➢ Blend

> ➢ Work the conditioner through your hair

> Start about ½ way between the scalp and the ends

> Working away from the head

> Do not put leave in conditioner on the roots of your hair – it will weight the hair down and cause it to look greasy more quickly

> ➢ Do not rinse

> ➢ Style as normal

These conditioner recipes also make a good deep treatment.

Using Daily Conditioner as a Deep Treatment

- ➤ Moisten a towel

- ➤ Heat in the microwave until warm

- ➤ Apply conditioner to clean, damp hair

- ➤ Wrap towel around head

- ➤ Wait until towel is cool to touch 3-5 minutes

- ➤ Rinse well

- ➤ Use weekly for best results

Hair Treatments

Sometimes your hair just needs some added boost. You can use your daily conditioner as a weekly deep treatment.

> ➤ Moisten a towel

> ➤ Heat for 30-60 seconds in the microwave

> ➤ Massage the daily conditioner of your choice into the hair

> ➤ Pile hair on top of your head

> ➤ Wrap in plastic

> ➤ Cover with the warm towel

> ➤ Let hair sit for 15-45 minutes

If you need a bit more, you can use one of these deep treatment packs.

Dry Hair Deep Moisture Pack

This is a nice deep conditioner that leaves your hair feeling silky soft. The conditioner leaves a weight behind, helping to minimize fly away, frizzy hair.

- ½   Mashed Avocado

- ½   Mashed Banana

Mash the fruit using a food processor, blender, or potato masher

- 1 tbsp   Coconut Oil

- 1 tbsp   Sesame Seed Oil

Warm Coconut Oil just until it is liquefied

Whip oils into fruit

When mixture is well blended apply to damp hair

Wrap hair in plastic

Allow mixture to sit for at least 30 minutes

Wash and style as usual

Damaged Hair Restoration Pack

This conditioner helps moisturize and strengthens damaged, overstressed hair.

- ➢ 2 tbsp   Gelatin Powder

- ➢ 2 tbsp   Colorless Henna Powder

- ➢ ¼ cup   Warm Water

Dissolve the Gelatin and Henna in the warm water

Whip in

- ➢ 1 tbsp   Meadowfoam Oil

- ➢ 1 tbsp   Rosehip Seed Oil

- ➢ 2 tbsp   Honey

When mixture is well blended apply to damp hair

Wrap hair in plastic

Allow mixture to sit for at least 30 minutes

Rinse hair and style as usual

Hair Conditioning and Thickening Treatment

This conditioner helps moisturize and strengthens damaged, overstressed hair.

- ➢ 2 tbsp   Gelatin Powder
- ➢ ¼ cup   Warm Water

Dissolve the Gelatin in the warm water

Whip in

- ➢ 1 tbsp   Wheat Protein Oil
- ➢ 4 tbsp   Champagne

When mixture is well blended apply to damp hair

Wrap hair in plastic

Allow mixture to sit for at least 30 minutes

Rinse hair and style as usual

Hydrating Hair Restoration Pack

I like to use a hydrating hair pack at least once a week to help keep my wavy hair in great shape. This pack works equally well on my daughter straight hair making it healthier, shinier, and beautiful!

> ➤ 2 tbsp   Gelatin Powder

> ➤ ¼ cup   Apple Juice or Pear or Berries

Heat your juice until it is just warm

Dissolve the Gelatin in the warm water

Whip in

> ➤ 1 tbsp   Paw Paw Oil

When mixture is well blended apply to damp hair

Wrap hair in plastic

Allow mixture to sit for at least 30 minutes

Rinse hair and style as usual

Fly Away Taming Pack

Whether your hair is naturally fly away or just needs a little help, this conditioning pack leaves it looking silky smooth and easy to style.

- ➢ 4 tbsp   Aloe Vera Gel

- ➢ 1 tbsp   Cocoa Butter

- ➢ 1 tsp   Wheat Germ Oil

- ➢ ¼ cup   Sugared Apple Juice

Blend ingredients until creamy smooth

When mixture is well blended apply to damp hair

Wrap hair in plastic

Allow mixture to sit for at least 30 minutes

Rinse hair and style as usual

Oily Hair Conditioning Pack

Even oily hair needs special treatment now and then. This helps to reduce excess oils and tone hair.

- ➢ ¼ cup   Yogurt - unflavored

- ➢ 2 tbsp   Almond Oil

- ➢ 3 tbsp   Orange Flower Water

Whip mixture until you have a smooth paste

When mixture is well blended apply to damp hair

Wrap hair in plastic

Allow mixture to sit for at least 30 minutes

Rinse hair and style as usual

Alternative Treatment Normal to Oily Hair

This makes a wonderful light conditioning treatment for normal to oily hair.

- ➢ ¼ cup   mashed cantaloupe

- ➢ 1 tsp   unflavored yogurt

Whip ingredients until creamy smooth.

When mixture is well blended apply to damp hair

Wrap hair in plastic

Allow mixture to sit for at least 30 minutes

Rinse hair and style as usual

Dandruff Control Treatment Pack

I love this treatment for soothing an itchy dry scalp whether dandruff is present or not. It is soothing and healing.

- ➢ 3 tsp   Jojoba Oil

- ➢ 1 tsp   Hemp Seed Oil

- ➢ 2 tsp   Vegetable Glycerin

- ➢ ½ tsp   Lavender Oil

Whip ingredients until creamy smooth.

When mixture is well blended apply to damp hair

Wrap hair in plastic

Allow mixture to sit for at least 30 minutes

Rinse hair and style as usual

Hair Loss Daily Scalp Massage

- ➢ 1 tsp   burdock root

- ➢ ¼ cup   warm water

Allow to steep 30 minutes

Strain roots   Can use Bur Oil in replacement

Add

- ➢ 1 tbsp   powdered ginger root

- ➢ 1 tbsp   powdered lemon balm

- ➢ 1 tbsp   birch bark oil

- ➢ 1 tbsp   black seed oil

- ➢ 1 tbsp   muira puama

- ➢ 1 tsp   lemon juice

- ➢ 20 drops   saw palmetto oil

Shake well

Massage into scalp 2-3x's daily

Do not use if you are on blood thinning medication, anti-coagulants or have a disorder related to blood
Do not use if you are pregnant or nursing
Do not use if you are unable to use aspirin
Not for use on children
For EXTERNAL use only

Fast Hair Growth Scalp / Root Spray

- ➢ 1 tsp   burdock root
- ➢ 2 tbsp   apache plume
- ➢ ½ cup   boiling water

Steep 30 minutes

Add

- ➢ 2 tbsp   Rosemary tincture

Massage into scalp 2-3 times daily

Do not use if you are pregnant or nursing

CHAPTER

6

Styling Aids

Once your hair is clean, conditioned, colored, and toned you need to style it. There is a vast array of styling products designed to do everything from boost shine to add volume.

The recipes in the previous chapters are designed to start achieving the goal of many of these styling products from the minute you begin your daily regimen.

As you use the shampoo, conditioners, and toners included in the guide you will begin to see less of a need for additional styling products.

By choosing the recipes designed for your care needs and customizing the ingredients to meet your specific hair type, you are creating healthier, better hair with each step.

Repairing Styling Gel

Sugar and proteins help to repair damaged hair and give it more body. This gel provides a nice thick appearance and light hold while promoting health.

- ➢ 1 cup   Distilled Water

- ➢ 1 packet   Unflavored Gelatin

- ➢ ½ tsp   Rosehip Seed Oil

Heat the water

Dissolve gelatin powder in water

Allow the mixture to cool

Store in a squeeze bottle or small tub

Use a small amount to set and style your hair

This mixture will be thinner at room temperature. If you prefer a thicker gel, store in the refrigerator.

Extra Hold Styling Gel

Gelatin gel makes a nice hold, but if you like a little extra control, this gel provides the same hair restoration and thickening while adding a little more hold. The fresh citrus scent gives a nice boost too!

- ➢ 1 cup   Unflavored Gelatin

- ➢ ½ cup   Grapefruit Juice

- ➢ ½ cup   Distilled Water

Heat the water and juice until it is hot, not boiling

Stir in the gelatin

Allow the mixture to cool

Add

- ➢ 1 tsp   Vegetable Glycerin

Store in a squeeze bottle or small tub

Use a small amount to set and style your hair

This mixture will be thinner at room temperature. If you prefer a thicker gel, store in the refrigerator.

Super Hold Styling Gel

This recipe makes a super control and thickening gel that is great for wet styles or hard to manage hair.

> ➢ 1 cup   Distilled Water

> ➢ ½ cup   Flax Seeds

Soak seeds in water for 15 minutes

Heat to boiling

Reduce heat and allow seeds to simmer an additional 5-10 minutes

Strain the seeds from the mixture

Allow the water to continue to simmer until the desired consistency is obtained

Allow mixture to cool

Add

> ➢ 1 tbsp   Grapefruit Seed Oil Extract

> ➢ 1 tsp   Essential Oil of Choice

Blend well

Store in a squeeze bottle or small tub

Use a small amount to set and style your hair

Hydrating Hair Gel

This is a nice light weight hair gel that gives good hold while attracting moisture. I like to use this on curly hair days but it works equally well for those with dry to normal hair regardless of the desired style.

> ➤ 1 cup   Distilled Water

> ➤ 1 package   Unflavored Gelatin

Heat the water and juice until it is hot, not boiling

Stir in the gelatin

Allow the mixture to cool

Add

> ➤ 1 tsp   Vegetable Glycerin

> ➤ 1 tsp   Paw Paw Oil

> ➤ 1 tsp   Honey

Blend Well

Store in a squeeze bottle or small tub

Use a small amount to set and style your hair

This mixture will be thinner at room temperature. If you prefer a thicker gel, store in the refrigerator.

Super Body Gel

If you have fine or thinning hair or need a lot of volume, a thicker styling agent that adds body, bounce, and shine to the hair.

- ½ cup   Distilled Water
- ½ cup   Flax Seeds

Soak seeds in water for 15 minutes

Heat to boiling

Reduce heat and allow seeds to simmer an additional 5-10 minutes

Strain the seeds from the mixture

Allow the water to continue to simmer until the desired consistency is obtained

Allow mixture to cool

Add

- ½ cup   Champagne or Sparkling Wine
- 1 tsp   Vegetable Glycerin
- 1 tsp   Wheat Protein Oil

Blend Well

Store in a squeeze bottle or small tub

Daily Detangler

This is an excellent detangler for children and adults alike. The recipe goes a long way so it is even perfect for sharing with others.

- ➤ 1 cup   Distilled water

- ➤ ¼ tsp   Vegetable Glycerin

- ➤ ¼ tsp   Grapefruit Seed Extract

- ➤ ¼ tsp   Aloe Vera Juice

- ➤ Essential Oil to Preference

Blend oils in a small pump bottle

Shake before each use

To use, spray on hair paying close attention to areas with excessive tangles.

Style as usual

Shine Serum

If you need or just love a little extra shine in your hair and want to add a bit of extra protection against styling, this serum is fantastic.

- ➢ 2 tbsp   Wheat Germ Oil

- ➢ 1 tbsp J   Jojoba Oil

- ➢ A few drops of your favorite essential oil

Blend oils in a small pump bottle

Shake before each use

To use, apply a small amount to the hair, staying away from the roots

Style as usual

Stimulating Shine Serum

My hair seems to grow so slowly at times. This serum is based on Rosemary. Rosemary is believed to stimulate hair growth. The serum gives my hair a lovely shine and who knows, maybe it does help my hair grow more quickly.

- ➢ 2 tbsp   Dried Rosemary
- ➢ 2 tbsp   Dried Nettle Leaves
- ➢ ¼ cup   Distilled Water

Heat water to boiling

Steep the rosemary & nettle leaves in the water

Strain herbs from water

Pour into a clean, dry container

- ➢ A few drops of Rosehip Seed Oil

Blend in a small pump bottle

Shake before each use

To use, apply a small amount to the hair, staying away from the roots

Style as usual

Texturizing Gel Spray

This is a nice texturizing spray you can use on the roots or shaft of your hair to promote body and help styling hold.

- ➢ 1 cup   Warm Water

- ➢ 1 tbsp   Sea Salt

Heat water

Dissolve salt in water

Add

- ➢ 1 tbsp   Aloe Oil

Blend in a small pump bottle

Shake before each use

To use, apply a small amount to the hair, staying away from the roots

Style as usual

Shine & Hold Spray

I like to use a spray whenever I can. This is a nice spray that gives hair a shiny look and mild hold.

- ¼ cup   Distilled Water
- 1 tbsp   Green Tea Leaves

Boil water

Steep teas until you have a very strong brew

Strain herbs

Allow mixture to cool

Add

- ¼ cup   Beer
- 1 tsp   Essential Oil of choice

Blend ingredients well

Pour into a clean pump style bottle

Shake well before use

To use, spray liberally from the roots to the ends of hair

Frizz Reducing Spray

I like to spritz my hair with this spray before styling. It helps reduce frizz. I also use it as a touch up on days with high humidity.

- ➢ 1 cup   Distilled Water

- ➢ 1 cup   Apple, Pear, or Berry Juice

- ➢ 2 tbsp   Wheat Germ Oil

Pour all of the ingredients into a clean spray bottle.

Shake well and lightly mist hair

Comb through to ends

Lemon Hair Spray for Normal to Oily Hair

This is a nice versatile spray that can be used as a root lift during styling or as a finishing spray. I like this for normal to lightly oily hair. If you have very dark hair, monitor your color to ensure the lemon zest is not causing unwanted lightening.

> - 1 cup   Boiling Water
>
> - 1   Lemon Peel – Finely Ground

Place the finely ground lemon peel in a glass bowl

Pour boiling water over the lemon

Cover and allow to steep 12-24 hours

Strain liquid into a clean pump bottle

Add

> - 1 tbsp   Rosewater
>
> - 3-4 drops Essential Oil if desired

Shake well and lightly mist hair

Can be used during styling or as a nice finish spray

Orange Hair Spray for Dry to Normal Hair

This is a nice versatile spray that can be used as a root lift during styling or as a finishing spray. I like this normal to slightly dry hair.

- ➤ 1 cup   Boiling Water

- ➤ 1   Orange Peel – Finely Ground

Place the finely ground orange peel in a glass bowl

Pour boiling water over the orange

Cover and allow to steep 12-24 hours

Strain liquid into a clean pump bottle

Add

- ➤ 1 tbsp   Witch Hazel

- ➤ 3-4 drops   Essential Oil if desired

Shake well and lightly mist hair

Can be used during styling or as a nice finish spray

Super Simple Spray

This is one of my favorite sprays. I like to scent it to suit the season and love that it is totally natural.

- ➤ 1 cup   Boiling Water

- ➤ 2 tbsp   White Sugar

Dissolve sugar in water mixture

Add

- ➤ 1 tsp   Aloe Vera Gel

- ➤ ½ tsp   Essential Oil of choice

Pour into a clean pump bottle

Shake well and lightly mist hair

Can be used during styling or as a nice finish spray

Wax Works Style Finishing Lotion

This is a nice hair cream that adds shine while helping to tame unruly hair.

- ➤ ¼ cup   Shea Butter

- ➤ 1 tsp   Coconut Oil

- ➤ 2 tbsp   Aloe Vera Gel

- ➤ 1 tsp   Almond Oil

- ➤ 1 tsp   Essential Oil of choice

Warm the shea butter and coconut oil until it is liquid form

Add remaining ingredients

Whip with a wire whisk until you have a creamy paste

Store in a clean, dry tub

To use, warm a small amount in the palm of you hand and work through dry hair

Moisture Infusing Finish Lotion

This is a nice hair cream that adds shine while infusing moisture throughout the day.

- ➤ 2 tbsp   Emulsifying Wax

- ➤ 1 tsp   Sesame Seed Oil

- ➤ 2 tbsp   Jojoba Oil

- ➤ 1 tsp   Almond Oil

- ➤ 1 tsp   Essential Oil of choice

Warm the wax until it is liquid form

Add remaining ingredients

Whip with a wire whisk until you have a creamy paste

Store in a clean, dry tub

To use, warm a SMALL amount in the palm of you hand and work through dry hair

This is an intensely moisturizing cream meant to be used in small quantities to help restore hairs natural health and vitality.

Extreme Moisture Cream

This cream may not work well for all hair types. It is an intense moisturizer meant to infuse moisture in to dry, damaged hair while helping give hair a nice texture.

- 2 tbsp   Olive Oil
- 1 tsp   Coconut Oil
- 2 tbsp   Sesame Seed Oil
- 1 tsp   Almond Oil
- 1 tsp   Emulsifying Wax
- 1 tsp   Essential Oil of choice

Whip with a wire whisk until you have a creamy paste

Store in a clean, dry tub

To use, warm a small amount in the palm of you hand and work through dry hair

CHAPTER

7

Nail Care

Many people go to great lengths to take care of their hands but often forget the nail area. The nails are a very important component to showing the world healthy looking and well cared for hands. The hands are a very expressive part of the body and are prominently displayed throughout your day.

Nails require care for both the cuticle areas and the nails themselves. Beyond the basic care I feel that there are few things I can do for myself that make me feel more pampered than a proper manicure. The recipes and treatments included in this section are effective for both fingernail manicures and toe nail manicures.

Manicure Basics

➤ Remove all traces of nail polish

➤ Soak your nails in warm water to soften the cuticles and rinse any residue left by polish removal and environmental factors

➤ Immediately apply cuticle cream to the softened cuticle areas

There are a variety of creams, both in this section and in the chapter titled lotions that work well on the cuticle area.

➤ Gently massage the cream into the cuticle area

➤ Push the cuticles back with a cotton swab or a cuticle stick

Never cut the cuticle areas as the rough areas left when they are cut can catch and tear.

➤ File your nails into the style that suits you best.

Some women prefer filing the nails into nice rounded tips while others prefer the flat edged look.

Whichever style suits your preferences, be certain you file the nails to a smooth finish to prevent the nails from cracking and chipping.

It is important to file the trim and file the nails to an even length. Regardless of the length you choose, a nice even distribution makes your hands appear better groomed and attractive.

After caring for the nails it is often beneficial to use a hand mask. This mask is similar to those you would use on your face and allow concurrent moisture of both your hands and nails at the same time.

If you choose not to use a mask treatment you should massage your entire hand and nail area with your favorite lotion or oils. Leave this lotion or oil massage on your hands as long as is feasible. This is an excellent before bed activity as it allows the full benefits of your lotion or oil to soak into your skin while you sleep providing deep conditioning.

Basic Henna Nail Strengthener

Strong nails are something each of us desire. Whether your nails are weakened due to your daily activities or are naturally weak because of hereditary this is an excellent strengthener that can go a long way toward providing the long, strong nails you desire. It is a quick recipe to create and a very easy product to use so I keep it around all the time and apply it a few times a week as part of my nail care maintenance.

- ➢ 1 tsp. **Colorless** Henna Powder

- ➢ ¾ cup Boiling Water

Dissolve the henna powder in the water stirring until well mixed.

Use only plastic or ceramic pans and utensils as henna powder can react poorly with metal.

If you desire a specific color or scent for your mixture you may add your favorite coloring agent or essential oils to the recipe.

Pour the solution into a clean container and seal tightly.

Soak your nails in this mixture 2-3 minutes 1-2 times daily for strong, healthy nails.

Allow the solution to dry on the nail area.

After the desired strength has been achieved you can apply the mixture with a cotton swab or cloth once or twice a week, allowing the solution to dry on the nails.

Be sure to use only colorless henna since henna is a dying product that can provide a semi-permanent stain to your nails.

Whitening Nail Soak

Stained nails are unattractive and embarrassing. Stains on the finger and nail areas can occur for a variety of reasons but can be easily eliminated. I do a lot of home renovations and my nails show the wear. Many of the products I use in our home repairs cause unsightly stains that take a long time to disappear. I use this solution every time I manicure.

- ½ tsp.　　　Sage

- ¼ cup　　　Water

Pour the water over the sage and allow to soak overnight.

Drain the leaves and add the water to the mixture below.

- 2 tbsp.　　　Rosewater

- 1 tsp.　　　Lemon Juice

Mix the ingredients until well blended.

The mixture will have a pretty scent but, if you desire a specific scent for your mixture you may add your favorite essential oils to the recipe.

Colorings are not recommended in nail bleach since the addition of color may alter the effect.

Store in a clean, tightly sealed container

Soak your nails in the mixture for 10 minutes twice daily until desired whitening has been achieved.

Whitening typically takes 3-7 days, depending on the amount of the stain.

I usually wipe the solution with a tissue and then follow with a moisturizing rub since my nails tend toward dry.

For a lighter application apply the mixture with a cotton swab and allow to dry on the nails.

Repeat this process twice daily until the desired bleaching effect has been achieved.

Always follow the whitening treatment with your favorite nail and cuticle balm or moisturizing hand lotion as the solution can be drying for your nails and dry nails will create another issue to address.

Nail Bleach

I like the whitening soak, but this solution is a great alternative because it gives a fresh scent and easy preparation process. The benefits of both products are very similar.

> ➢ 2 tsp.   Orange Flower Water

> ➢ ¼ tsp.   Lemon Juice

Mix the orange flower water and the lemon juice in a clean container.

Seal tightly.

The mixture will have a pretty scent but, if you desire a specific scent for your mixture you may add your favorite essential oils to the recipe.

Colorings are not recommended in nail bleach since the addition of color may alter the effect.

Apply using a cotton swab.

Allow the mixture to dry for approximately 10-15 minutes and repeat the process as needed up to 2-3 times daily until desired results have been achieved.

Always follow the treatment with a moisturizing nail/cuticle balm or a moisturizing hand lotion since the bleach product can be very drying.

Nail Strengthening/Hardening Balm

Sometimes colorless henna can be difficult to locate in the town where I live. I use this recipe as a quick replacement for my regular nail strengthening soak whenever we run short of the henna. The benefits of both recipes are similar and it is a matter of preference which you use.

- ➤ 1 tbsp.   Water

- ➤ 1 tsp.   Honey

- ➤ 1 tsp.   Alum Powder

Dissolve the alum powder in the water.

Use ceramic or plastic pans and utensils as alum powder may react with metal.

Use only USP Grade for Cosmetic use Alum Powder.

Add the honey and stir until a light gel is formed.

If you desire a specific color or fragrance you may add your favorite colorant or essential oils to the recipe.

Spoon into your favorite container

Apply to nails using a cotton swab.

Allow the mixture to dry on the nails approximately 10-15 minutes.

Repeat this process 2-3 times daily until nail strength has been obtained.

After nails have reached the desired strength apply this mixture 1 time daily to maintain the new nail strength.

Always follow nail strengthening products with a moisturizing nail/cuticle balm or a moisturizing hand lotion since these products can be drying to the nail and cuticle areas.

Cuticle Balm

This is an excellent moisturizing and protective balm that you can use daily. I like this one following any nail care treatment that dries my nails since lanolin and apricot kernel oil are very easily absorbed and provide a lovely shine. The coco butter provides a protective film that helps keep the environment from further drying my nails.

- ¼ cup   Grated Coca Butter

- ½ tsp.   Lanolin

- 3 tbsp.   Apricot Kernel Oil

Mix all ingredients in a microwave safe dish and microwave on medium heat for approximately 30 seconds until the mixture is creamy.

Stir all ingredients until well blended – approximately 1 minute.

If you desire a specific color or fragrance you may add your favorite colorant or essential oils to the recipe.

Allow the mixture to cool approximately 2-3 hours. You may place the container in the refrigerator to speed the cooling process.

Gently massage mixture into cuticles as often as desired to achieve soft, attractive looking cuticles.

Nail/Cuticle Strengthening Balm

I love to use this product for moisturizing and strengthening benefits all in one step. I use this whenever the weather is colder and my nails and cuticles really suffer or just when I am short on time and cannot perform multiple step care to obtain strength and moisture.

- ➢ 2 tsp.   Castor Oil

- ➢ 1 tsp.   Vitamin E Oil

- ➢ 2 tbsp.   Orange Flower Water

Stir all ingredients until well blended.

Approximately 1 minute.

Massage mixture into cuticles two times daily until soft and healthy cuticles have been achieved.

To maintain this appearance continue to use once or twice a week during normal conditions – more frequently if your hands have been roughened or the climatic conditions are unduly harsh.

This balm also works very well for extremely rough/dry hands.

Massage mixture into hands in the same manner as you used for the cuticle until softened skin has been obtained.

Softening Cuticle Balm

Everyone suffers from ragged and hard cuticles at some point. This recipe is a great solution since it is easily absorbed and provides excellent softening benefits.

- ➢ 2 tsp.   Almond Oil

- ➢ ½ tsp.   Wheat Germ Oil

- ➢ 2 tsp.   Petroleum Jelly

Stir all ingredients until well blended. Approximately 1 minute.

If you desire a specific color or fragrance you may add your favorite colorant or essential oils to the recipe.

Massage mixture into cuticles two times daily until soft and healthy cuticles have been achieved.

To maintain this appearance continue to use once or twice a week during normal conditions – more frequently if your hands have been roughened or the climatic conditions are unduly harsh.

This balm also works very well for extremely rough/dry hands.

Massage mixture into hands in the same manner as you used for the cuticle until softened skin has been obtained.

You may wish to enlarge the recipe if you plan to use this as a hand balm as well as a cuticle balm.

Anti-Aging and Healing Hand and Cuticle Balm

This is a great lotion I use on my hands nearly every day. Hands in my family seem to dry out and age more quickly so hand care is especially important to me. This product contains known anti-aging properties as well as excellent moisturizing and protective ingredients. The components also work very well for the daily care of the cuticle combining both steps in one. During the busy workweek I often find that I have to skip or combine steps to ensure that every part is taken care of in the correct manner. This combination product helps save time while delivering incredible benefits.

> ➢ 1 tsp.   Aluminum Sulfate

> ➢ 2 tbsp.   Lanolin Oil

> ➢ 1 tsp.   Glycerin

> ➢ 1 tbsp.   Wheat Germ Oil

> ➢ 4 tbsp.   Aloe Vera Gel

Mix the Aluminum Sulfate with the oils until well blended.

Be sure to use only USP Grade for Cosmetic use Aluminum Sulfate.

Mix ingredients in a plastic or ceramic container.

Add the remaining ingredients and heat in a microwave safe dish in the microwave on medium heat approximately 20 seconds.

Stir well. If you desire a specific color or fragrance you may add your favorite colorant or essential oils to the recipe.

Pour into clean container. Allow mixture to cool and massage into your hands and cuticles as often as desired.

Vitamin E Lotion

This is another great product for massaging into both the hands and cuticles. The recipe includes some well known anti-aging ingredients as well as anti-oxidants, which are believed to slow the effects of aging. I love this recipe because it provides deep penetrating moisture to my hands and cuticles while providing a nice healthy glow to my nail area.

- 1 tsp.   Vitamin E Oil
- 2 tbsp.   Orange Flower Water
- 1 tsp   Stearic Acid
- ¼ cup   Soft Cocoa Butter
- 1 tsp   Glycerin
- 1 tsp   Honey

Place cocoa butter, glycerin and honey in a plastic or ceramic microwave safe dish.

Heats on medium approximately 20 seconds until the ingredients liquefy.

Dissolve stearic acid in solution and add Vitamin E Oil and Orange Flower Water.

Stir well.

If you desire a specific color or fragrance you may add your favorite colorant or essential oils to the recipe.

Pour the solution into a clean container.

Seal tightly and apply to hands and cuticles as often as desired.

CHAPTER 7

Lip Care

Many people forget that proper care of their lips is a vital part of the beauty regimen. Often lipsticks or lip treatments are chosen based upon the color or staying power of the item rather than the content. Lips can age and become unattractive unless proper care is taken to maintain a healthy and youthful appearance.

An important point to remember is that unlike the rest of your skin, lips do not contain any oil glands. This makes it especially important to use products that infuse the lips with moisture while providing a protective coating to prevent drying.

Making lip care products is a very simple process. Often combining only one or two ingredients can make a fantastic product customized toward your skin type and lip care needs. Most people hesitate to create their own lip care products because of their inability to obtain just the right color. There are many natural dye products that can be used to create the perfect color for all of your lip products, lipsticks, lip glosses, even chap sticks! In addition to these natural dye products, there are many chemical colorants that can be blended to obtain just the right shade.

Natural Lip Care Product Colorants

Alkanet Root:
red root, which comes from a tree and aids in the dying of products.

This is an excellent base for your lipstick colorant as it is a basic red and could be modified to present a brighter shade or darkened through the use of purple-red beet juice or brown-red henna and tea products.

Beet Powder
Beet Juice:
a lovely purple red color which can be altered or adjusted depending on the shade desired.

This is an easily obtained dye that is a by-product of the beets.

This is one of my favorite colorants because the juice gives the product a light sweet flavor.

Carmine:
red pigment derived from dried cochineal.

This is another excellent base for your lipstick colorant.

It provides a glowing red shade that can be modified to suit your exact color needs by adding other products to obtain a purple or brown cast.

Cranberry Juice
Creates a gentler form of the red glow found in some other dyes and colorants.

Grape Juice

Stains from grape juice are a common concern around the house. Now, by mixing the lovely dark shade of pure grape juice with other desired colors you can obtain a dye that will provide a lovely purple red glow to your lips

This is another of my favorite colorants because all of the flavor of the grapes will be present every time you apply your gloss or lipstick!

Henna

Most people are unaware that henna powder comes in a variety of shades and that the longer you let the henna soak in the liquid form the darker the shade will become.

This is an excellent colorant for those who desire a darker color or brown red effect.

This color may cause a dyed look to the lips and should be carefully monitored to ensure a semi-permanent lip appearance is not created unless the color is a look you desire.

The use of henna for colorant provides the added benefit of a lip protection ingredient. Henna forms a protective coating which is excellent for the maintenance of your lip condition during harsh climatic conditions.

Tea

For those who prefer a tan or brown shade to their lipstick the addition of tea can provide a lovely color ranging from a light golden glow found in chamomile to a darker brown shade using teas such as orange pekoe.

Experiment with the various teas you currently use paying close attention to the color of the water. To create stronger tones simply steep your tea in a smaller amount of water for longer periods.

The liquid colorants can be used in place of many of the liquids in the following recipes to generate the color you desire.

In addition to color, creating your own lip care products provides another exceptional opportunity for customization. Most people have specific flavorings that they prefer and benefits they require. By creating your own lip care products you have the opportunity to add flavorings that suit you likes and moods.

Moisture Infusing Lip Stick

A good moisturizing lip stick is an essential part of any beauty care regimen. Most of us don't realize how much moisture our lips lose on a daily basis or even that moisture is essential to healthy lips making a moisture infusing stick a must have rather than a beauty extra. This is a nice stick I like to carry with me at all times. I apply a little whenever my lips feel a bit dry. In addition to providing a fantastic protective moisturizer for my lips it looks great!

- ¼ cup   Grated Beeswax

- 1 tbsp.   Lanolin

- 1 tsp.   Petroleum Jelly

- 1 tbsp.   Apricot Kernel Oil

- 2 tbsp.   Favorite Juice

Pear/apple/cherry/berry juices all provide a moisture attraction. Choose the color juice that is best for your needs.

Additional dyes may be added to alter the color of the stick or the juice may be left out if preferred.

The juice will also provide a pleasant flavoring without the need for additional additives.

Place the grated beeswax, lanolin and petroleum jelly in a microwave safe dish and microwave on medium for approximately 45 seconds.

Remove the mixture from the microwave and allow to cool slightly.

Stir in the apricot kernel oil and preferred juice until well mixed.

Pour the solution in a greased container and allow to cool.

Approximately 12-16 hours until solution is hardened. Placing the container in the refrigerator may speed the process.

Cut the hardened product into sticks and apply.

Basic Beeswax Lipstick

I like to use beeswax as my lipstick base. Beeswax is gentle, has many healing and anti-bacterial properties, and makes a firm lipstick that holds up well over time.

- ➢ ¼ cup   Grated Beeswax

- ➢ 3 tbsp.   Apricot Kernel Oil

- ➢ 2 tbsp.   Grated Cocoa Butter

- ➢ 1 tbsp.   Coconut Oil

- ➢ 2 tbsp.   Lecithin

- ➢ 1   Vitamin C Tablet

Mix oils, beeswax and cocoa butter in microwave safe dish.

Microwave on medium approximately 1 minute

When mixture is a golden brown liquid, add the crushed Vitamin C tablet and stir until dissolved.

Allow mixture to cool slightly and stir in your favorite colorant and flavorings as desired. These are not a necessary additive to the mixture.

Pour mixture into a greased container and allow to cool and harden.

Approximately 12-16 hours. Placing the container in the refrigerator may speed the process.

Cut the hardened mixture into sticks and apply.

Makes approximately 5 ¼ inch x 2 inch sticks

Protective Lip Stick
Perfect for harsh climatic conditions

We live a very active outdoor life and there are times in both the summer and winter months when my lips need some extra care and attention. This is an excellent basic stick for harsher climates and it works especially well when my lips become chapped. I like to separate the mixture before hardening to add a variety of flavorings and colors.

- ➢ 4 tbsp.   Grated Coca Butter   (stick)

- ➢ 1 tbsp.   Zinc Oxide

- ➢ 1 tsp.   Apricot Kernel Oil

- ➢ 1 tsp.   Honey

Place grated cocoa butter in a microwave safe dish and microwave on medium heat for approximately 20 seconds until the mixture is a pasty liquid.

Stir in remaining ingredients until well mixed.

Be sure to use only USP Grade for Cosmetic use Zinc Oxide.

Add colorant or flavors as desired.

Pour mixture into a greased container and allow to harden. Approximately 12-16 hours. Mixture may be placed into the refrigerator to speed the process.

Cut mixture into sticks and apply.

These sticks will be slightly softer than the basic lipstick recipe.

Makes approximately 5 ¼ inch x 2 inch sticks

Healing Chapped Lip Stick

This is an especially popular mixture for the guys. Many of the men in my family neglect their lips until they become chapped. Then they want an instant cure. I like to keep a few of these around, especially during the colder months.

- ¼ cup   Grated Beeswax

- 3 tbsp.   Apricot Kernel Oil

- 2 tbsp.   Grated Cocoa Butter

- 1 tbsp.   Aloe Vera Gel

- 1 tsp.   Zinc Oxide

- 1 tsp.   Honey

Combine all the ingredients in a microwave safe dish.

Use the solid form cocoa butter for best results.

Be sure to use only USP Grade for Cosmetic use Zinc Oxide.

Microwave on medium heat approximately 45 seconds until the mixture is a soft creamy liquid.

Stir gently to combine all ingredients.

Add your favorite colorant or flavorings if desired.

Pour the mixture into a greased container and allow to cool.

Approximately 12-16 hours. Placing the container in the refrigerator may speed the cooling process.

Cut the hardened mixture into sticks and apply.

Makes approximately 5 ¼ inch x 2 inch sticks

Almond Oil Lip Gloss

Sometimes a nice glossy look is a must have. When I want a glossy look or just to add some moisture to my lips I use this instead of some of the other products designed to promote healing.

- ➤ 1 tsp.   Grated Beeswax

- ➤ 1 tsp.   Grated Cocoa Butter (stick)

- ➤ 1 tsp.   Almond Oil

- ➤ 1 tsp.   Apricot Kernel Oil

Mix all ingredients in a microwave safe dish and microwave on medium heat for approximately 20 seconds.

A thick mixture should form.

Gently stir until all ingredients are well blended.

Add your favorite colorant or flavoring.

Pour into a clean lip gloss container and allow to cool.

Mixture will stay somewhat soft for easy fingertip application.

Moisture Locking Lip Gloss

This is a fantastic finish stick. It gives the lips a nice shiny look and locks in moisture. I like to carry this in my purse for freshening throughout the day.

- ➢ 1 tbsp.   Coconut Oil

- ➢ 1 tbsp.   Petroleum Jelly

- ➢ 1 tbsp.   Apricot Kernel Oil

- ➢ 1 tsp.   Stearic Acid

Add favorite colorant or flavoring as desired.

Combine all ingredients in bowl and whip until well mixed approximately 1 minute.

Spoon mixture into lip-gloss container and apply with fingertip or applicator.

For a more liquid from lip-gloss leave out the stearic acid

Liquid can be applied with a brush or sponge applicator.

Thicker Lip Gloss

This recipe creates a much thicker gloss that retains its shine much longer than some of the others. I really love this whenever I know I have hours and hours to go before I can refresh my make up.

- ➤ 10   Psyllium Seeds
- ➤ ½ cup   Boiling Water

Pour boiling water over psyllium seeds

Allow to soak for 6-12 hours depending on the thickness desired

The longer the seeds soak the thicker the final results will become.

Strain liquid from seeds and discard the seeds.

- ➤ ¼ cup   pear juice (apple, cherry, berry)
- ➤ 1   Vitamin C Tablet

Crush the Vitamin C tablet and dissolve into the juice mixture.

Slowly add juice mixture to the psyllium seed gel stirring thoroughly.

The mixture will form a very heavy gloss that will provide a high shine and a protective moisturizing base for your lip care.

This gloss is much thicker than usual and you will want to experiment with soak time and the amount of juice added to the seed gel to obtain the best texture for your needs.

The juices you have chosen will provide color, flavor and fragrance to your product, but if you desire a specific color, flavor or fragrance you may add your favorite flavorings, coloring or essential oils to the mixture.

Chapped Lip Balm

Our lips get very chapped when the seasons change. We keep chapped lip balm ready for each member of the family.

- ➢ 10   Alder Leaves

- ➢ ¼ cup   Boiling Water

Pours boiling water over leaves and allow to set for approximately 6 hours until a tea substance is obtained.

- ➢ 1 tsp.   Aloe Vera Gel

- ➢ 3 tbsp.   Petroleum Jelly

- ➢ 3 tbsp.   Stearic Acid

Add alder leaves liquid to the other ingredients stirring gently.

The result will be a very soft balm, which can be rubbed into lips for relief from cracking and irritation.

For a thicker end result use more stearic acid and for a softer result use less stearic acid.

Add desired colors or flavorings.

Spoon into a clean gloss container and seal tightly.

To apply use fingertip or applicator to apply a light coat to your lips

Lip Blemish Sticks

At times we all get a pimple, ulcer or other blemish around our lip area. This is an excellent product that will help promote faster healing of these eruptions while aiding in the prevention of additional blemishes.

- ➢ 4 tbsp.   Grated Beeswax

- ➢ 1 tsp.   Honey

- ➢ 2 tbsp.   Apricot Kernel Oil

- ➢ 1 tsp.   Powdered Bloodwort

- ➢ 1   Vitamin C Tablet

Place beeswax, honey and oil in a microwave safe dish and heat on medium approximately 25 seconds.

Dissolve powdered bloodwort and crushed Vitamin C tablet in the heated solution and mix well.

If you desire a specific color, flavor or fragrance you may add your favorite flavorings, coloring or essential oils to the mixture.

Pour the mixture into a greased pan and allow to harden approximately 12-16 hours. You may place the container in the refrigerator for faster results.

Cut the hardened mixture into sticks and apply as needed.

Appendix A Ingredient List

All natural make up and personal care products have become 'the thing' for many people. Whether from a desire to reduce chemical usage, reduce expenses, address specific issues better than the mass market products or just live a more natural life, more and more people I speak with are making their own cleaners, make-up and beauty products.

My family has used 'natural' products for years. My mother and grandmother both had skin and allergy issues and passed many home cleaning, personal care, and other product ideas down to my daughter and I. My daughter was born with the same sensitive skin and had the added issue of being a chemical reactive asthmatic.

I have posted many video and recipe instructions for the products that we use and enjoy the most. However, there are many reasons that people want to make their own natural products and your needs may not be the same as ours. There are also many combinations of product components that we have not yet tried. The following pages list some of the most commonly used elements and their supposed properties and effects.

Before you begin using the included ingredient lists, please remember that the properties and effects shown for each ingredient has not been fully proven and in many cases endorsed by the FDA or AMA. Whenever I am aware of a particular approval or endorsement, have included the information. All of this information has been gathered over years of use, chats with other people, and trial and error research. Please use your care and your own common sense when trying any of the included ingredients.

Enjoy!

Acacia	Powdered Acacia is used as a binding agent for lotions, ointments, and other liquids to semi-solids
	Soluble in cold water
	Improves texture of semi-solid preparations
Acetamide MEA	Used as a stabilizer
AHA	Alpha Hydroxyl Acids are acids extracted from fruit, sugar and vegan lactic acid
	Will dissolve dead cells
	Mild peeling and moisturizing
	Use 1 – 5% in creams and gels
	DO NOT use around eyes or on sensitive skin
Almond Oil	Easily absorbed
	Natural astringent and emollient characteristics
	Softens and conditions the skin and hair
	Used in lotions, treatments, and ointments For all skin types
	Alleviate itchy skin conditions

Alkanet Root	Red root that comes from a tree
	Aids in the dying of products

Allantoin Powder	Protects against harsher components of recipes
	Helps stimulate growth of tissues
	Use .5 to 2% in creams
	Inhibits allergic responses
	Dissolve in a little cold water and then add while product is less than 40 degrees
	Classified by the Food and Drug Administration (FDA) Over-The-Counter (OTC) Topical Analgesic review Panel as a Category I (safe and effective) active ingredient skin protect, at use-levels of 0.5 - 2.0%. FDA approved applications include minor cuts, scrapes, burns, sunburn, fever blisters, diaper rash and chaffed, chapped, cracked or wind burned skin and lips. It is a skin protect for use in creams, lotions, lip products, shaving creams, suntan products, scalp healing products, and baby products Reference FDA Release

Almond Butter	Excellent spreadability
	Adds moisturizing attributes to creams, lotions, bar soaps, hair care, sun care, balms and oils

Almond Oil	Contains Oleic Acid, fatty acids, sterolins and Vitamin E
	Nearly odorless
	Skin nutrition
	Similar to skins natural oil
	Natural emollient
	Tames fly away
	For all skin & hair types
Aloe, Aloe Vera	Soothing
	Anti-inflammatory
	Antibacterial
	Treatment of acne
	Highly emollient
	Believed to stimulate collagen synthesis and skin regeneration
	Leaf is rubbed on dry hair tame fly away ends
	Oil promotes healing and replaces lost moisture
	Improves hydration
	Cuticle – heals, smoothes, softens

Aloe Butter	Extract of aloe in a coconut base
	Solid at room temp but melts on the skin
	Lotions & creams 3-5%, Balms 5-100%, Conditioners 2-5%
Aloe Oil	Add healing properties to recipes without bacterial or mold growth (5-10%)
Aloe Wood	Used in skin tonic mixtures
	May have pigment restoration qualities
Alpha Hydroxyl Acids(AHA)	Mild acids that remove the outer layer of dull skin
	Creates a rejuvenated appearance
	Contains glycolic, lactic, malic, citric and tartaric acids that are mild acids used to remove the outer layer of dull skin
	From citrus fruits, apples and grapes
	Glycolic acid is found in sugar cane
	Lactic acid is found in milk
	The FDA now requires that any product containing AHA's have the following warning statement: This product contains an alpha hydroxyl acid (AHA) that may increase your skin's sensitivity to the sun and particularly the possibility of sunburn. Use a sunscreen and limit sun exposure while using this product and for a week afterwards Reference: FDA Release

Aluminum Sulfate

Acts as an antiseptic

Aids in stopping bleeding

Aids in tightening skin

Tightening agent for year rounds use in aging products

*** Purchase ONLY cosmetic grade

Amino Acids - Oat

Oat Amino Acids penetrate easily

Humectants, soothing, itch reliever, moisturizer

Deposit protective film on hair – smoothing and moisturizing

Amino Acids - Silk

Body uses as a building block

Penetrates well

Ammonium Lauryl Sulphate

Shampoo base derived from coconuts

Creates lather

Cleanses hair while separating strands to give volume

Promotes spreading of product

Andiroba Oil

The oil contains myristic acid

Help minimize the growth of the pigment producing cells that cause age spots

Apache Plume

Root and bark are boiled as with tea

Used as a hair tonic to promote growth

Apple Juice

From the apple

Rich in pectin

Apricot Kernel Oil

From apricot pits

Similar to natural oils

Moisture without oily film

Rich in Vitamin A

Extremely nourishing

Emollient

Softer and smoother feel

Easily absorbed by the hair and skin

Infuses moisture into the hair and skin

Argan Oil

Helps increase squalene

Rich in Vitamin E and Fatty Acids

Absorbs Quickly

Strengthens Brittle Hair & Nails

Believed to replace lost moisture

Anti-aging effect when massaged into the skin

Arrowroot

Minor anesthetic qualities

Excellent balm for irritated scalp

Thickening and stabilizing agent

Ascorbyl Palmitate

Palmitic acid ester - Vitamin C Ester

Salt of ascorbic acid

Used as a preservative and antioxidant

Believed to remove the free radicals that cells produce

Asphodelus

Used as part of a topical ointment or cream to fade freckles, age spots, scar tissue, and excess skin pigmentation

Avocado

From the fruit of avocados

Used often as a moisturizer

Protects hair and skin in hot, dry climates

Rich in oils

Sunscreen properties

NOT for oily skin

Year round uses especially in summer

Nail – Cuticle care

Rich in Vitamins B, E, and K

Deep moisture treatments

Avocado Butter	Soft greenish butter
	Mild odor but excellent melting properties
	Softens and moisturizes
Avocado Oil	Rich, heavy, penetrating oil
	Vitamin A, C, D, E
	NOT for oily skin
	May repel UV rays
	DILUTE with other oils to minimize thickness
Baking Soda	Clarifying agent
	Softens water to enable cleaning agents to work better
Bananas	Mashed fruit of the banana
	Rich in oils
	Non-irritating
	Excellent for all hair types
	High potassium content makes it difficult for bacteria to survive
	Rich in Vitamin A
Bay Rum	Stimulates scalp to encourage hair growth

Bearsfoot Root/ Yellow Leaf Cup root	Used as an ointment Shampoo component to treat scalp conditions such as dandruff
Beer	Beer is an excellent product base for hair rinse or finishing products The sugar base and protein components of the beer act as a thickening agent and can be used as a hair rinse or combed through hair before styling to provide a fuller, lustrous look to the hair Aroma fades as beer dries Hair – especially for thinning or fine hair Thickens, adds shine, and adds bounce Rinse or styling agent Year round use
Beet-root Powder Beet Juice	Purple red color Tastes sweet
Benzoin	Use benzoin resin in external skin applications heal cuts, sooth inflammation of rough cracked skin Used as a preservative in cosmetics and a fixative for perfume

Beta carotene

Vitamin A

Found in plants and many animal tissues

Has an orange pigment and is used as a coloring agent in several cosmetics

Excessive beta carotene in the blood can lead to a yellow-red pigmentation of the skin

Birch bark

Helps halt hair loss

Black Seed Oil

Nutrating oil

Contains fatty oils, vitamins & minerals

May aid in preventing hair loss

Contains amino acids that help to strengthen and nourish the hair

May combat alopecia when included in a topical scalp treatment

Borage

High gamma linolenic acid GLA – Vitamin for skin

Humectants

Skin disorders like psoriasis and eczema, and sun damaged or aged skin

Regenerating and stimulating for all skin types

Borax

Used as a preservative and texturizer

Excellent cleanser that is mild and allows the creation of cleansing products without drying the skin and hair

Adds foaming effect to soaps

** Borax Powder (Sodium Borate – natural source of cosmetic grade borax that does not contain surfactants and detergents. Acts as an emulsifier

Burdock Root Oil

Also known as Bur Oil

Improves hair strength, shine & body

May help prevent hair loss

Soothing – eases dandruff & scalp itching

Promotes hair strength, shine, and body

Boil ½ tsp of root in 1 cup of water and allow to steep for 30 minutes. Up to 3 x's daily.

Burdock root tea can be used alone or as a part of a skin wash to help combat acne

Cajeput

Astringent oil

Good for oily skin

Helps clear eczema

Calendula Oil

Targets oil or Marigold Oil

Antiseptic, antifungal, anti-inflammatory

Healing, soothing – all skin types

Can relieve acne

Camphor

Antibacterial, astringent

Combat oily skin and acne

Cantaloupe

Light hair conditioner for oily hair

Carmine

Red pigment derived from dried cochineal

Excellent dye for lipsticks

Carrot Oil

Rich in beta carotene, Vitamin A & E

Balance moisture in skin and conditions hair

Revitalizes and tones and nourishes skin

Easily absorbed

Helps balance both oily and dry complexions

Heals damaged skin

Helps aged skin

Castile Soap

Made from olive oil

Extremely mild, liquid with water-like consistency

Can be used on both hair and skin

Provides gentle cleansing without drying

Leaves a soft, moist feel when rinsed

Castor Oil

Hard shiny oil that acts as a barrier agent and protector

Found in many cosmetics

Cedar wood

Sedative, astringent, antiseptic

Used to treat oily skin and scalp

Relieve itching, psoriasis, eczema,

High concentrations will irritate the skin

Good insect repellent - mosquitoes, moths, woodworms, leeches and rats

Centaury

Helps clear blemishes

Softens the skin

Said to remove freckles, age, & hyper-pigmentation

Cetearyl Alcohol	Emulsifying wax produced from mixture of fatty alcohols
	Forms a barrier film to keep moisture from evaporating
	Give hair and skin a velvety feeling
	Used to add body and compatibility to hair
Cetearyl Glycoside	Made of glucose and cetearyl alcohol
	Helps hair retain moisture
	Creates velvety feeling
Champagne	Can also use sparkling wine
	Rich in sugars and proteins
	Acts much like beer and thickens hair while providing body and bounce.
	Hair – Styling lotion, thickening rinse, wet/dry gel
	Promotes tissue regeneration
	Used to treat dermatitis, minor skin irritation and inflammation
	Bleaches fine, light hair
Clary Sage	Treatment for oily hair and skin
	Dandruff control treatment
	Treats wrinkles

Chlorophyll	Derived from the leaves of green plant
	Promotes healing
	Excellent deodorizer
Cinnamon	Darkens hair
Citric Acid	Preservative
	Extends products shelf life
	Helps products retain texture and guards against appearance loss
	Blends easily
	Contains Alpha Hydroxyl
Cleavers	Used as a skin wash
	Improve complexion
	Treats skin disorders
	Used as a dandruff relief hair rinse
Cocomphcaroxy-glycinate	From coconuts
	Works with sodium lauryl sulphate
	Makes shampoo milder on skin and hair

Cocomide DEA	From coconuts
	Makes bubbles smaller so that foam is thicker and richer
	Fatty acid from coconut oil and glycerin
	Used in shampoos, conditioners and shower gels as a thickener and foamier
Cocoamidopropyl Betaine	A coconut oil compound
	Used as an emulsifier, thickener, foam booster, and conditioner
Cocoa Butter	Soften and lubricate
	Cuticles – soften/protects
	Hair – styling tames hair on ends – similar to wax works
	Prevents drying and chapping
	100% COCOA BUTTER ONLY
Coconut Oil	From coconuts
	Provides exceptional protective layer to hair, skin, lips, and cuticles
	Locks in moisture
	Straighten hair while locking in moisture
	Emollient
	Treats dry, damaged hair
	Suitable for all skin and hair

Penetrates into the deeper layers of the skin to helping to keep connective tissues strong and supple

Easily absorbed

Helps to reduce the appearance of fine lines and wrinkles

Aid in exfoliating the outer layer of dead skin cells

Cod Liver Oil   Source of EPA and DHA and Vitamin A&D

Collagen   Pseudo Collagen

Derived from yeast

Mimics the action of collagen and confers moisture

Binding

Adds body and shine to hair

Pour. 5 to 10% into product while under 40 degrees

Copaiba   Effective in fighting dandruff

Relieve inflammation

Help heal athlete's foot, eczema and psoriasis,

Heals damaged skin with minimal scarring

Cornflower	Astringent
	Added to shampoo to treat eczema of the scalp
Cornstarch	From corn ground fine – white powder
	Replaces many powder ingredients
	Excellent thickening agent
	Absorbs Moisture & Oils
	Leaves hair extra shiny
Cottonseed Oil	Rich in Vitamin E
Cranberry Seed Oil	Skin, hair, lips and baby care
	Contributes to lipid barrier protection
	Assists in moisture retention
Cypress	Reduces excess oils in skin and hair care products
	Tightens skin
	Refine the appearance of pores
	Reduces excess sweating in overly oily hair
Diazolidinyl Urea	Preservative

Distilled Water

Water with all minerals, bacteria and other substances removed

Egg Yolks

Contains lecithin - a natural emulsifier and preservative

Rick in protein

Aids in creating shiny, thicker hair

Hair – deep conditioner, hair thickening agent

NOT moisturizing

Excellent for oily hair

Elderberry

Darkens gray hair

Emulsifier

Used to create bond between water and oil

Critical in lotions and creams

Makes a fluid cream and lotion without separation

Nice end texture

Mixes two opposing liquids making it an excellent additive for many products

Evening Primrose Oil

Nutrating oil

Contains fatty oils, vitamins & minerals

May aid in preventing hair loss

AMA says makes skin softer, smoother, reduces roughness, cracking and irritation
Reference AMA Release

Flax Oil

Richest source of alpha linolenic acid

Reduces trans epidermal water loss from skin

Fumitory

Treatment for eczema and other eruptions of the skin

Helps removing freckles

Gelatin

Derived from animal collagen

Beneficial to hair and nails

Contains high levels of sugar and protein

Help repair damaged hair and promote body

Setting agent or deep conditioner for hair

Can be used as a rub for nails

Germall Plus

Preservative

Liquid / water soluble

Highly effective

Geranium

Mature and troubled skin care

Creates a radiant glow

Ginkgo

Improves circulation aiding in combating hair loss

Glycerin	Natural humectants (attracts and holds moisture)
	Pulls oxygen from air and brings it to hair
	Very gentle even for sensitive skin
	Year round use for hair
	Perfect for all weather
	Vegetable glycerin – natural emollient
	Hypoallergenic
Gotu kola	Contains asiaticoside
	Works to stimulate skin repair
	Strengthens skin, hair, nails, and connective tissue
Grapefruit Juice	High in citric acid
	Contains natural sugars, which help thicken and hold hair in place
	OILY hair only
	Hair – Oily hair styling agent, Hair Spray
Grapefruit Oil	Hair growth
	Antiseptic, Astringent
	Oily hair only

Grapefruit Seed Oil	Made from dried ground seeds and pulp of grapefruit
	Natural preservative
	Antiseptic, anti bacterial
	Stabilizing for most products
	Combined with glycerin in many items
Rapeseed Oil	Odorless oil
	Base for many creams, lotions and as a carrier oil
	Does not leave greasy feeling
	Non-allergenic
	Oleic, linolec, palmitric and stearic acids
	Emollient and toning to all skin types
Green Tea Extract	From the leaves of the plan dried, cured, extracted into ethyl alcohol
	Astringent
	Mixes well with both oil and water based products
Guar Gum	Made from the ground seed tissue of plants
	Used as a thickener
	Has 5 to 8 times the thickening properties of starch
Hazelnut Oil	High in Vitamin E
	Easily absorbed into hair

Hempseed Oil

Highly absorbent, soothing

Especially rich oil

Said to stimulate cell growth

High in linolenic acid

Emollient

AMA – skin feel softer, smoother, reduce roughness, cracking and irritation
May retard fine wrinkles of aging
hair care products, hemp seed oil increases elasticity, manageability, and shine
Reference AMA

Henna Leaves

From henna plants these leaves are resinous

Provides a protective coating for hair, lips, nails and skin

Can be used colored in tanning products and hair dyes

Locks in moisture

Protects from elements

*** Henna is a dye – colorless leaves are available.

Purchase only 100% henna at most drugstores and pharmacies

Nails – strengthening agent

Locks in moisture

Excellent for dry, damaged, weak nails

Hair – provides a thicker, lustrous appearance for hair

Locks in moisture, protects and strengths

Hibiscus Flowers	Provides red highlights to light or dark hair
Honey	Derived from the nectar of flowers and plants and created by bees as a by-product of honeycomb creation

98% sugar and 2% enzymes

Full of Vitamins and minerals

Has a stimulating and toning effect

Natural humectants

High potassium content inhibits bacteria growth

Excellent component for moisturizing formulations

The DARKER the honey the better the effect care because the dark honey contains more minerals.

Attracts moisture and helps lock it in place

Hydrates

*** Do not use honey in child care products or those who commonly come into contact with children as honey can be harmful to the very young

*** Natural preservative

Lips/nails – harsh climatic conditions – attracts and holds moisture

Hair – humectants which attracts and holds moisture. Assist in curly hair curl hold

Hair – lightens slightly – use molasses for darker hair care products

Honey Powder

Full of Vitamins and minerals

Natural humectants

High potassium content inhibits bacteria growth

Excellent component for moisturizing formulations

*** Do not use honey in child care products or those who commonly come into contact with children as honey can be harmful to the very young

*** Natural preservative

Imidazolidinyl Urea

Preservative

Immortelle

Stimulate the production of new skin cells

Mature skin products

Jasmine

Used in ointments for dry sensitive skin

Jojoba Oil

Actually a liquid wax

Very similar to body's natural oil making it easily absorbed

Perfect for any moisturizing agent

Will solidify if kept cold

Mimics collagen

Year round use for hair, nails, skin and lips

Moisture – hair and skin easily absorbed

Natural preservative

Carrier oil

Scalp cleanser for hair

(application) 11%

Hypoallergenic and pure

Kokum Butter

Naturally white and very smooth

Emollient properties

Hard / solid – melts on contact

Lotions and creams 1-3%, balms 5-100%, conditioners 1-3%

Kukui Nut Oil

Expressed from the nuts, and is light yellow with an amber tint

Aids in softening and restructuring

Easily absorbed

Highly penetrating

Hydrate and soften

Lanolin Oil

From glands of sheep

Waxy feel substance

Acts as moisturizing agent for skin, lips, nails

Setting lotion for hair

Helps absorb and retain moisture

May penetrate the skin and hair follicles

Deep treatment base

Deep conditioning

Emollient – soothing and softening

Lavender Oil

From lavender flowers

Antiseptic – germ killing properties

Enhances highlights in dark hair and darkens lighter hair

Astringent - ideal for oily and combination skin

Lauramide DEA

From coconut and palm kernel oils

Prevents harsh stripping action of shampoo by coating hair and giving bounce

Lauryl Betaine

From coconut and palm kernel oils

Boost foam in shampoo

Lecithin

Derived from egg yolks , soybeans, and corn

A natural emollient

Allow special proteins to penetrate better

Attracts water from the air and holds hydration in place – skin and hair.

Can get in powder form

Emulsifier and thickening agent

Lemon Balm

Baldness Prevention

Lemon / Citrus

Derived from the juice of citrus fruits

Anti-bacterial

Creates highlights in light hair when used in small quantity in a hair rinse

Hair – year round use as a clarifying agent to reduce the build up of gels and oils

*** Remember lightening effect – dark hair use Baking Soda

Lemongrass

Astringent, anti-septic, anti-infectious, antifungal

Good for oily hair

Reduces excessive sweating and enlarged pores

Great for oily skin and hair

Lemon Oil

Balances sebum (skin oil)

Increases shine and growth of hair and nails

Astringent

Lightens hair

Brighten dull complexions

Gentle cleanser for oily skin and hair

Acne treatments

Add after any steps that require heat

Do not expose to high temperatures

Macadamia Nut Oil	Similar to sebum (natural oil)
	Absorbs well
	Emollient and soother
Magnesium Sulfate	Water softener
Magnesium Stearate	From ester of magnesium and stearic acid
	Odorless fine white powder
	Soluble in warm alcohol
	Insoluble but dispersible in water and oils
	Provides opacity, texture & consistency
Mayonnaise	Created from eggs, oil and vinegar
	Moisturizing agent for hair
	Oil and eggs provide nourishment for hair and skin
	The vinegar provides a clarifying effect to hair and skin
	Can be used as a deep moisturizing agent
Meadow foam Seed	Adds shine and moisture to hair and scalp
	Helps dry and brittle hair
	Cuticle repair, body oils, shaving creams

Menthol Paraben	Non-toxic, nonirritating
	Preservative
	Stable in most ingredients – water soluble
Milk, Goat	Lactose leaves the hair and skin feeling silky smooth
	Softening cleanser
	Hydrates
	Alpha hydroxyl treatments = lactic acid (milk) + citric acid, glycolic, malic and tartaric acids
Milk, Powdered	Lactose leaves the hair and skin feeling silky smooth
	Excellent softening cleanser
	Hydrates
	Alpha hydroxyl treatments = lactic acid (milk) + citric acid, glycolic, malic and tartaric acids.
Mint Leaves	Rich in iron
	Natural energizer
	Kills bacteria
Nettle Leaves / Root	Stimulates hair growth
	Improve condition of scalp
	Contains chlorophyll and silicone - silicone assists in hair and nail strength

Oats	Oatmeal
	Soothing skin treatment - dry skin, sunburns, eczema, psoriasis
Olive Leaf	Relieve itchy scalp
Olive Oil	Nutritive and stable
	Superior penetrating power
	Acidic and antioxidant
	Cleaning agent shampoo/conditioner
Optiphen	Liquid preservative
	Add at anytime during creation
Orange Flower Water	Derived from orange blossoms
	Astringent and cleanser
	Hair – remove gel and build-up
Orange Peel	Use the entire orange peel (white and orange)
	Mild abrasive combined with the natural solvent of orange oils
	Vitamin rich
Orrisroot	Derived from root of white iris
	Used as fixative for perfumes and powders
	Retains aromas

Palm Kernel Oil

Similar to coconut oil

Lathers well

Papaya Paw Paw

Natural softener for hair and skin

Creates a velvety feel

Patchouli

Heals dry and itching skin

Pear Juice

Good source of sorbitol – humectants

Attracts moisture

Provides a smooth texture

Assists in curl creation

Apples, cherries, plums and berries have the same effect

Pineapple Juice

Contains bromalain, a protein digesting enzyme

Removes dead cells, surface dirt, and oils

Hair – clarifying treatment for oily hair

Polysorbate 20

Vicious oily liquid from lauric acid

Emulsifier

Common component of coconut oil

Allows water to penetrate more easily

Pomegranate	Use only the seeds, not the whole fruit
	Deep penetrating oil
	High in flavinoids
	Good for dry, devitalized skin
	Aids in moisturizing skin, preventing and reducing the appearance of wrinkles
	Used to treat dry skin, eczema, psoriasis
Proteins	Add gloss, body and luster to hair
	Plant proteins have excellent skin compatibility
Propyl Glycol	From lactic acid, glucose or seaweed
	Most common moisture carrying agent in cosmetics
	Moisturizes better than glycerin
	Gives product better absorption and spreadability
	AMA says – safe in cosmetics
Propyl Paraben	Widely used in cosmetics
	Preservative against bacteria and fungus
	Paraben is neutral – non irritating, non-sensitizing
Psyllium Seeds	From plants
	These create a very thick gel
	Surrounds hair and helps hold a set

Tames fly away hair and for structured styles

Pygeum	Used with Saw Palmetto & Stinging Nettle Root for hair loss treatments
Red Raspberry Oil	UV absorptive properties – all three levels
Rhubarb	Lightens hair
	Mix w/ shampoo for color treatment
Rose / Rose Water	Astringent skin care wash
	Speeds healing
Rosehip Seed Oil	Derived from the ripened fruit of a hybrid rosebush
	Strengthens hair shaft
	AMA says it makes skin feel softer and smoother, reduce roughness, cracking and irritation. Possibly retard the fine wrinkles of aging Reference AMA Release
Rosemary Oil	Antioxidant
	More stable than Vitamin E for products and creams
	Helps stop products from going rancid
	Preservative
	Tames fly away hair
	Brings out warmth in darker hair
	Stimulates the scalp

Slows hair loss

Speeds hair growth

Astringent

Anti-bacterial

Safflower Oil

Highest Linoleic Acid

Moisturizing

Treats dry and damaged skin

Soothing to skin

Contains two colorants – yellow & red

Used for dyeing silk

Mixed with finely-powdered was used to create 'rouge.'

Pale yellow oils contain proteins, minerals, vitamins

Good for all skin types

Sage

Darkening Hair Dye - Especially for gray hair

Stimulating to the scalp

Softens & shines hair

Invigorates scalp

Dries perspiration – lessens body odor

Oils are antiseptic and antibiotic

Sal Butter	Stable
	Extremely emollient
	Prevents drying
	Directly applied in solid state or mixed
Sandalwood	Relieves inflammation and itching
	Helps dry and dehydrated skin
	Mild astringent
	Helps with acne and other inflammatory skin conditions
	Good for oily skin
Saw Palmetto	Saw palmetto inhibits dihydotestosterone (DHT), - enzyme that is associated with male pattern baldness
	May halt hair loss
	Stimulates healthy hair growth
Sea Buckthorn	Combat wrinkles
	Good for severe dryness
	Used as part of treatment for premature aging
	Repairs, conditions, and heals damaged skin
	Acne treatment
	Will stain skin, surfaces and clothing.
	Apply evenly to skin surfaces

Dilute prior to use

Use at room temperature

Sea Silk

Marine vegetable

Provides protein enrichment

Creates silky feeling

Protective, moisturizing film

Soothes the scalp

2-3% into product while under 40 degrees

Seaweed

Contains carregenall which is an emulsifier

Sesame Oil

From sesame seeds

Sunscreen

One of the deepest natural oils

Shea butter

Rich is vitamins A, E, and F

Protects the skin from free radicals

Helps prevent lines and wrinkles

Moisturizes dry, heat-damaged, over processed hair.

Hydrates hair

Humectants - draws moisture into the hair

Coats the shaft to make hair soft

Forms breathable, water resistant film

Compatible with all hair types

Solid

Melts at skin temp

Use as little heat as possible to reduce granules

3-5% lotions and creams, 5-100% balms, 3-6% bar soaps, 2-5% conditioners

Slippery Elm

Emollient

Slightly astringent

Soapwort

Base ingredient in liquid soap, shampoo, & conditioner

Not lathering

Gives hair & skin a slippery feel

Sodium Hydroxymethylglycinate

Antimicrobial

Used in VERY low concentrations

Preservative for products – can be used in place of TEA

Active regardless of the other ingredients used in the recipe

Amino acid – helps penetration

Sodium Lauryl Sulfoacetate

Free flowing white powder

Use in cream and paste shampoos, cleansing creams, and bars

Provides foaming and viscosity

Milder to the skin than ethoxylated alcohol sulfates such as Sodium Lauryl Sulfate

Hard water stable

Used to replace soap

3% concentration

Sodium Laureth

Shampoo base from palm and coconut oils

Foams and cleanses

Sorbitol

Humectants

Gives smooth feel to hair

Used instead of glycerin in many recipes

Occurs in ripe berries, cherries, plums, pears, apples, seaweed, and algae

Humectrant and a binder

Gives hair and skin a velvety feel

Soyamidopropl Betaine

Compound from soybean oil & alcohol

Used as an emulsifier, thickener, foam booster and conditioner

Spearmint

May help to control excessive hair growth in women

Used in facial steam to help cleanse and tighten pores

Squalane	Increases spreadability of lotions
	Colorless, transparent and fragrance free
Stearalkonium Chloride	Ammonium compound
	Adds shine to hair
	Improves ability to comb hair
	Conditioning ingredient that forms a protective coating on the cuticle
	Retards tangling
	Assist with manageability
Stearic Acid	From animal fats – white, waxy powder
	Melted to clear liquid it provides a thick, stiff texture to creams and aids in keeping oils and waters together
	Emulsifier (primary purpose – most common use)
	Known for the pearly or waxy feel it adds to creams
	Ultimately has a cooling effect when applied to skin
Strawberry	Has a natural PH like skin
	Mild, effective treatment for all skin types
	Nourishing as a soap or lotion component

Strawberry Leaves

Bleaching action

High in Vitamin C

Acidic astringent

Mild anti septic

Sunflower Oil

Moisturizes and regenerates surface cells

Vitamin A & E rich

Protects skin from ultraviolet light

Prevents cell damage from free radicals

Wrinkle fighting

Tamanu nut

Healing to serious skin problems

Used on scrapes, cuts, burns, insect bites and stings, acne, acne scars, psoriasis, diabetic sores, anal fissures, sunburn, dry or scaly skin, blisters, eczema, diaper rash, herpes sores

Treats dry, irritated, mature skin

Promotes healthy, clear, blemish-free skin

Helps clear acne

Fades acne scars

Antimicrobial, antibacterial and anti-fungal

Effective on scabies, ringworm, and athletes foot, jock itch

Tincture

Herbal preparations make with alcohol

Gives longer shelf life to product

Tincture of Benzoin

From gum resin

Used as a preservative

Emulsifier

Some antiseptic properties

Titanium Dioxide

Cream that blocks the suns rays

Use micro-encapsulated kind for easier mixing

White, odorless powder pigment of crystalline structure

High refractive index

Water resistant

Provides long-term UV-protection

Insoluble but dispersible in water and oils

Triethanlamine (TEA)

Emulsifier that works with stearic acid

Vinegar

Derived from fermented fruit juices

Aids in removing reside from the hair

Acts as a clarifying agent when mixed with water

Vinegar is a STRONG substance that can be damaging when applied directly

MUST BE DILUTED

Vitamin A	Beta Carotene
	Causes orange color in cosmetics
	Vitamin A
	Antioxidant - aids removing free radicals
	Encourages collagen production - causes the skin to plump out
	*** Monitor use carefully as too much can cause damage
Vitamin B	Cumulative conditioning effects in hair products with extended, regular use
	Absorbed by the hair to protect form atmospheric conditions
Vitamin C	Found in many fruits and vegetables
	Acts as a preservative and anti-oxidant
Vitamin E	Natural preservative
	Emollient
	AMA – make skin softer, smoother, reduces roughness, cracking and irritation
	May retard signs of aging
Vodka	Derived from potato and grains
	Used in cosmetics for hair
	Acts as a solvent
	Product Base

Watercress	Juice has a mild acid that contains iron, minerals and phosphorus
	Clarifying agent for oily hair – removes soap residue and oils
Water Dock Root	Used in ointment or shampoo to treat scalp conditions – dandruff
Watermelon Oil	Dissolves Sebum

WAXES

Beeswax	Derived from the secretions of bees when they are forming honeycombs
	Forms a protective barrier on the hair
	Provides a guard against environmental factors
	Anti-bacterial
	Tames fly-away hair
	Used in straightening agents
	Repels moisture – limits frizz or curl
	Cuticles – provides protection, sooths frayed torn cuticles
	Emulsifier and stiffener
Candelilla Wax	From candelilla plant, a desert shrub native to New Mexico and Texas
	Thickener (can be used to replace beeswax)

Carnauba Wax

From leaves of Brazilian wax palm tree

Melting point is 181 degrees

Extremely hard wax for hard set recipes

Emulsifying Wax

Polawax

Plant based

Emulsifier – used to create bond between water and oil

Good in lotions and creams

Makes a fluid cream and lotion without separation

Nice end texture

Jasmine Wax

Floral wax from jasmine distillation

Fragrant thickener

Wheat Germ Oil

High in Vitamin A, B1, D, lecithin, protein and fatty acids

Very high Vitamin E

Very emollient – needs mixed to remove sticky

Preservative

Wheat Protein

Hydrolyzed (turned partly into water) = nitrogen carrying

Beneficial to hair = protein

Add gloss, body and luster to hair

Deposits a protective film on the that is smoothing and moisturizing

Witch Hazel

Astringent that can be used on irritated skin

Calms itchy uncomfortable skin

Xanthan Gum

Natural sugar

Gel Thickener

Thickens and stabilizes products but difficult to work with because it does not dissolve in water

Yarrow Root

Contains azulens

Anti-inflammatory

Reduces effect of unbroken blemishes

Yogurt

Made from fermented milk combined with bacteria

Skin softener

Zinc Oxide

*** Purchase only USP grade intended for cosmetic use

Antibacterial, antiseptic, astringent

Protective

Can be used as a sun screen

Encourages healing

White pigment

Appendix
B
Recipe
Locator

167

www.ingramcontent.com/pod-product-compliance
Lightning Source LLC
Chambersburg PA
CBHW081826280526
45789CB00007B/2357